Weight Loss
Confidential
Journal

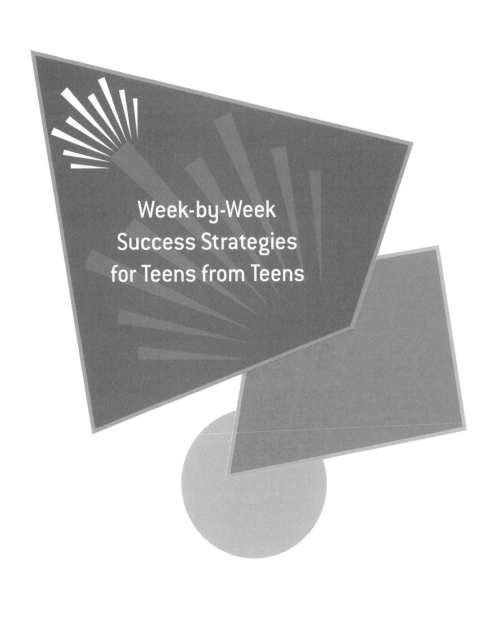

Week-by-Week
Success Strategies
for Teens from Teens

Weight Loss Confidential Journal

A companion book to
WEIGHT LOSS CONFIDENTIAL:
HOW TEENS LOSE WEIGHT AND KEEP IT OFF
— AND WHAT THEY WISH PARENTS KNEW

Anne M. Fletcher, M.S., R.D.

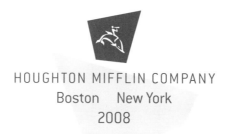

HOUGHTON MIFFLIN COMPANY
Boston   New York
2008

For information about permission to reproduce selections from
this book, write to Permissions, Houghton Mifflin Company,
215 Park Avenue South, New York, New York 10003.

Visit our Web site: www.houghtonmifflinbooks.com.

LIBRARY OF CONGRESS CATALOGING-IN-PUBLICATION DATA

Fletcher, Anne M.
Weight loss confidential journal : week-by-week success strategies for teens from teens /
by Anne M. Fletcher.
p. cm.
ISBN-13: 978-0-618-43372-8
ISBN-10: 0-618-43372-4
1. Weight loss—Juvenile literature. 2. Reducing diets—Juvenile literature.
3. Teenagers—Nutrition—Juvenile literature. I. Title.
RM222.2.F5372 2007
613.2'5—dc22   2007009417

Book design by Anne Chalmers
Typefaces: Minion, Conduit, August-Light

Printed in the United States of America
MP 10 9 8 7 6 5 4 3 2 1

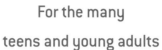

For the many
teens and young adults
who, in their willingness to help others,
shared their stories for *Weight Loss Confidential*
and *Weight Loss Confidential Journal*

Author's Note

This book is designed for teens who are truly overweight, a condition that should be determined by a physician.

You should consult a physician before following the advice or guidelines in *Weight Loss Confidential Journal.* This is particularly important if you have a medical condition such as diabetes or high blood pressure. A registered dietitian's counsel is advised as well. If you're overweight and trying to reach a healthier weight, you should be monitored regularly by your physician to make sure you're healthy and growing properly. If you have an eating disorder or think you might have one, you should speak to a physician and/or a licensed mental health professional to determine whether the advice in this book is appropriate for you. This advice is also important if you are experiencing psychological distress, such as depression.

Before starting any weight loss plan, diet, or exercise regimen, you should seek the permission and supervision of your physician, who might want to run some tests to make sure your weight problem is not caused by a medical condition.

All the teens in this book have given their permission to share information about their weight histories. For those under the age of 18, their parents have given their permission as well. Most of the names have been changed to protect the teens' privacy. Sometimes the teens' remarks were edited for clarity or were paraphrased. Some of the facts in this book may have changed since the information was gathered.

Weight Loss Confidential Journal

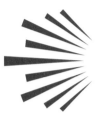

"I lost 152 pounds, and it's been 12 years since I started the journey. But it all begins with a choice. Something makes you think, 'Wow, I deserve so much more than this' and 'I can do anything I want.' Once this 'aha' moment arrives, the remaining journey continues to be filled with choices. You have a choice each day about whether to exercise, eat properly, take care of yourself mentally — or accept that there are going to be setbacks. You have a choice each day to better yourself."

—Amber M.

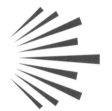

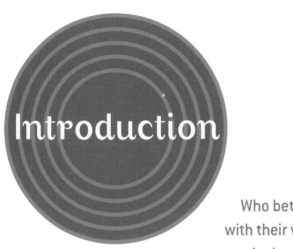
Introduction

Who better to help teens
with their weight than other
teens who have "been there"?

Weight Loss Confidential Journal takes inspirations, advice, and helpful strategies from teens who used to be overweight, then lost weight in healthy ways, and puts their insights into a format that can help you make changes — one week at a time. It also gives you a place to write down what you eat, keep track of your progress, and write about how you're feeling as you take steps to get to a healthier weight. (You can go through the weeks in any order you want.)

Take the case of Wes G., who became very overweight when he was a teenager. By the end of 11th grade, he weighed 270 pounds. Even though he was 6'1" at the time and big-boned, he was way too heavy and not very happy about it. However, Wes managed to lose 65 pounds when he was a senior in high school and grew an inch. He's kept the weight off for more than 3 years. Although he wound up using strategies for healthy weight loss that he learned while growing up, he had to lose weight his way, in his own time — and he had to want to do it for himself.

When Wes was 13, he was going through the cafeteria line at a summer academic camp and noticed that a thin boy in front of him ordered a salad with dressing on the side and took a diet soda instead of a regular one. When Wes asked him why, the kid pulled out a photo of himself when he was at least 40 pounds heavier and said, "Everyone in my family eats like a slob, and I didn't want to be like them!" Even though he didn't lose weight until years later, Wes now says, "I remember thinking,

'If this kid with overweight parents and negative influences could do it, so can I.'" Wes and the boy started sharing weight loss tips — something neither one had ever been able to do before.

By using this journal, you'll be able to benefit from the insights and experiences of many teens, like Wes, who used to be overweight.

Do It *Your* Way

If you feel discouraged because everyone in your family is overweight or you've tried to lose weight before and then gained it back, don't give up. Most of the 104 teens interviewed for *Weight Loss Confidential* come from families with other overweight people, many had been heavy for a long time, and most had lost weight and gained it back at least once before finally succeeding. The teens interviewed lost, on average, 58 pounds, and three quarters of them lost 30 pounds or more. And they've been successful at keeping their weight off. Although some of the teens didn't lose that much weight, they grew in height, which made their weight and height "match" better. In other words, they "grew into" their weight.

"There were so many times when I felt like trying was pointless, but I finally did it. And if I could do it, then anyone can."

— Sandra D.

As the teens' stories show, there's no single program, diet, or workout routine that works for everyone. Ally S., who lost 56 pounds 5 years ago, says, "Find a diet and exercise plan that's right for *you*. If you enjoy the foods and activities, you're more likely to stick to a healthy lifestyle." She's right. With the help of your physician and parents, you need to find a way to slim down that suits you as an individual. (At the back of the book, you'll find a healthy weight management food plan.)

Kelly D., who tried to lose weight three or four times before succeeding, says it's good to experiment. "Keep trying new things until you find something that works," she advises. In general, a program should emphasize a variety of healthy food choices, physical activity, and changes in habits that you can live with for a lifetime. It's best if you can find a program specifically designed for teens, such as one at a local hospital or university. If you slim down on your own or are using a commercial program, check with your physician and, ideally, a registered dietitian to make sure you're losing weight in a healthy way.

The teens mentioned exercise most often as their most important weight loss strategy. Next came remarks about eating sensibly or having more healthy foods. And whether they slimmed down on their own or went to a program, virtually all the teens used a combination of different strategies — typically, eating fewer fatty foods, getting more exercise, watching calories, downsizing portions, snacking less often, and/or cutting back on food in general.

"If you starve yourself and then start eating again, you actually gain back more weight than you had before."
— McKenzie K.

Over and over, the teens stressed the importance of using healthy strategies — not extreme measures, such as skipping meals, taking diet pills, or following fad diets. Many went to programs that gave them guidance on how to lose weight safely.

As you go through the journal, keep in mind that it was a combination of strategies that helped these teens slim down. They didn't do everything all at once. As David G. says, "Losing weight is a journey that needs to be taken a day at a time."

Setting Goals You Can Reach

This journal gives you a place to record your goals for each week. We're not talking about weight goals here but, rather, about setting one or two manageable weekly goals having to do with changes in your eating or exercise habits that will ultimately help you reach your long-term goal of a healthier weight. Jack F. says, "Remind yourself numerous times throughout the day of your goals and how you're attaining them."

Xavier L. says, "It's really important to have small goals." It's helpful to focus less on the scale and more on your eating and exercise habits. For instance, you can decide how often you walk home from school instead of getting a ride or choose frozen yogurt over a hot fudge sundae. That way, weighing yourself once a week can become a sort of "reality check" to see how things are going.

One of the ways to shift your focus toward habits you can directly control is to set realistic targets. Unrealistic goals can make you feel discouraged and set you up for failure.

TAKE BABY STEPS TOWARD A HEALTHIER WEIGHT. Margaret G. lost about 25 pounds between the ages of 16 and 21. Gradually, she stopped adding gravy to foods, ate fewer sweets, took smaller portions, and continued to be active in sports, bike riding, and a dance group.

A realistic "baby step" goal for exercise might be going for a 20-minute walk every other day as opposed to running a mile a day, which probably isn't realistic if you're not in shape. Gradually, walk a bit more.

DON'T SET "NEVER," "ALWAYS," OR "GIVING UP" GOALS. Wes G. says, "I often got discouraged when I failed to meet lofty goals, like 'I'm giving up ice cream.' I succeeded when I used landmarks: 'I'll only have ice cream once a week.' I was pleased with my step-by-step progress."

MAKE YOUR GOALS SPECIFIC, SO THERE'S SOMETHING YOU CAN MEASURE OR COUNT. It's hard to measure progress toward vague goals such as "I need to eat more fruits and vegetables" or "I'm going to get into shape." But you can really tell how well you're doing with specific goals like "I'll eat breakfast at least 5 days this week," "I'll have one fruit or vegetable with every meal and snack," or "I'll go to the gym and lift weights for half an hour, 3 times a week."

The journal can help you set goals. For instance, in Week 16: Cut Your "Seat Time," your goal might be to reduce your TV watching, video game playing, and IM time to 2 hours or less each day so that you can be more active.

> "I decided to break down the scary lifestyle change into smaller, more manageable changes. Changing my perspective made losing weight seem more realistic and doable."
>
> — Paula D.

Planning for Things That Might Trip You Up

Under the goals section for each week, you'll find space to write things that might get in the way of your weight progress in the week ahead. You can also use the space to plan how to cope with these obstacles. For instance, you might be going to a party on Saturday that will be tempting because of all the snack foods. So write that down under "Things that might trip me up." Then, under "How I plan to deal with them," you might write, "I will pick three things that I really like and keep the portion sizes small."

Here are some other examples:

Things that might trip me up:	How I plan to deal with them:
Tuesday: class trip	I'll pack my own lunch.
Friday: sleepover at a friend's	Before going, I'll eat a light supper so
	I'm not starving/bring my own diet
	soda/have one treat at the sleepover.

Don't be hard on yourself if your "plan" doesn't work — use the situation to figure out a better way to handle things the next time. At the end of each week, you can record the strategies that worked.

> "Exercise suppresses my appetite for junk and allows me flexibility in how much I eat."
>
> — Jeana S.

The Power of Exercise

Jorgey W. says that the most important thing she does to keep off the more than 100 pounds she's lost is "exercise at least every other day." Her exercise includes 3-mile runs on a treadmill, plus lifting weights 4 days a week.

Exercise can help when you're feeling down or stressed out, as Sandra D. notes: "Once I started getting into the exercise routine, it became almost like meditation for me. During my workout, I started to reflect on things going on in my life and used my workout as a time to relieve any stress." Exercise may even help you do better in school, as Marie P. found when she started working out: "Not only did I feel better, but I ended up getting better grades and having more energy."

What Kind of Exercise and How Much?

Although some of the teens participated in organized sports, most didn't become star athletes or marathon runners. From hip-hop and belly dancing to in-line skating and running, they figured out how to turn moving their bodies into having a good time. Eleanor F. advises, "Make exercise fun. To make myself interested at first, I'd just dance around my room and work up a sweat." Katie S. says, "I always exercise with the music pumped up. It gets the adrenaline flowing and makes the time fly by."

> "Start walking, even if it's just a little at first."
>
> — Erin C.

Most of the teens did more than one kind of activity, which helps keep exercise from becoming boring. Many of them switched off between strength training and aerobic exercise, which is probably the best combination for weight control. Aerobic exercise includes activities such as brisk walking, jogging, fast dancing, swimming laps, step aerobics, playing tennis, and bicycling. Strength training* can be done by using free weights, resistance bands, and/or equipment such as Cybex or Nautilus weight machines. (Pushups and abdominal crunches are other forms of strength training.) Other activities that count as exercise include playing around outdoors, chores like raking and mowing, walking to school, and actively participating in physical education classes.

Whether or not you're overweight, you're supposed to get at least

---

*Experts recommend doing strength training (8 to 10 different exercises) 2 or 3 days a week, with one full day of rest between workouts so that the muscles have time to recover. (Or upper and lower body muscles can be worked on alternate days.) Ideally, if you're new to strength training, it's wise to start with the help of a trainer who has experience with young people. The trainer should have a college degree in exercise physiology and/or certification through a national program such as the American College of Sports Medicine or the National Strength and Conditioning Association.

60 minutes a day of moderate to vigorous activity. But if you've been inactive, work your way up to that gradually.

Any exercise is better than none, as Jorgey W. points out: "If you're too tired to work out, just do some of your favorite exercise. Then at least you got some exercise in."

Contrary to popular opinion, the "no pain, no gain" philosophy just isn't true. If exercise hurts, it's not okay. Pain or discomfort in a bone, joint, or muscle is a signal to stop exercising and consult a doctor. Exercise should also be stopped if you experience chest discomfort or pain, dizziness, severe headache, or any other unusual symptoms. Such problems call for medical attention. If you're overweight and you want to start vigorous exercise, get a doctor's okay first.

Don't be alarmed if you gain a bit of weight when you first start working out, particularly with strength training, since muscle weighs more than fat. If you continue to burn more calories than you're eating, you'll eventually start losing weight again, making up for the slight amount of weight you gained from developing bigger muscles.

The teens made exercise a priority. Sandra D. says, "I forced myself to go to the gym regularly so it became part of my weekly routine. I started going for about an hour 3 times a week. And the more I went, the longer I stayed and the more often I went."

> Kristy C. says, "If I treat my exercise time like any other class, it reinforces my perception of it as important."

The second page for each week of the journal has a place for you to schedule your exercise. Give some thought to the week ahead and the time of day when you will exercise, then try to be specific about what kind of exercise you'll do and for how long. (It's okay to build in some days off from exercise. Many of the teens didn't exercise every single day.) Each day, fill in "What I actually did" in the journal to see whether you're following through on your plan or whether you need to adjust things.

Why Keeping Track Works

"Keeping track of what I ate and the minutes I exercised in a daily planner gave me a way to see my progress," says Jon M., who lost 82 pounds at 16. "It kept me motivated and helped me make sure I was honest with myself. Sometimes I still look at my old records to remember what I've done, and it reminds me of how far I've come." Studies suggest that kids who keep track of what they eat are more likely to lose weight than those who don't keep track.

"When I began exercising, I used to feel people were thinking, 'Oh, look at that fat kid.' Now I realize that other people who are working out respect it when someone who's overweight sticks to a workout plan."
— Tyler D.

It's ideal if you can write things down shortly after you've eaten them, but that's not always practical. Jon M. says he usually did that before he went to bed. "Doing that once a day let me think of it more as record keeping for my body — just like I'd make sure my bank account was in order. By writing things down, I could evaluate my day to be sure I was making good choices." Once a week, he'd weigh himself and write that down too.

Ally S. found that keeping a diary helped her see patterns that were tripping her up. She explains, "If I didn't lose any weight, I might look back on the week and see that I'd eaten out a lot. Or if I saw that I didn't work out much, it explained why my clothes were fitting differently."

Keeping a Daily Diary

When you record what you eat and drink, don't forget between-meal or evening snacks. For cooked foods, note how they're prepared — for instance, fried, broiled, or with a sauce. And don't forget "extras" that have calories, like butter, mayonnaise, and salad dressing. (There's no need to keep track of things that have few or no calories, like diet soda, water, black tea or coffee, or sugar-free gum.) It's also important to write down the amount of each item you eat or drink. To get an idea of amounts and portion sizes, it's helpful to measure foods, at least for a while.

You may find it useful to fill out the "Hunger" column to tune in to whether you're eating something because of true biological hunger. (You don't need to do this for every item — just overall, for meals and snacks.) In the "Calories/Other" column, you can keep track of anything extra you want to pay attention to, such as calories or fat grams. Noting any emotions you were feeling when you were eating ("stressed out," "worried," "lonely," "angry," "bored") will help you recognize when you're eating for emotional reasons.

In the "Exercise/Physical activities" space, don't forget to count informal activities like throwing a Frisbee for your dog, walking to school, or parking the car at a distance from the store to do some extra walking.

The "Plan for tomorrow" space encourages you to think ahead. For instance, if you didn't get up early enough for breakfast one day, your "plan for tomorrow" might be to "set the alarm for 6:45 so I have time for breakfast."

Under "Today's successes/Random thoughts," you can jot down more about how your day went. Get into the habit of patting yourself on the back for at least one daily achievement or positive step. Your successes might include getting up early enough to have a bowl of oatmeal before school, ordering a grilled chicken sandwich instead of a double cheeseburger, or calling a friend rather than raiding the fridge.

> "What the scale tells you does not define your health or your worth."
> — Tyler D.

Weekly Review

When you get to the Review of My Week page, consider the things that really helped and reward yourself for the goals that you met. No, not with food, but with something like going to a movie, buying a CD, or getting your nails done. If you didn't attain a goal, don't beat yourself up — just ask yourself what got in the way and whether you need to change the goal to make it more realistic.

Although you can record your current weight, it's important to remember the many other ways to recognize your progress. As Tyler D. says, "If you continue to maintain a healthy lifestyle, then what the scale tells you does not really define your health or your worth. Weight is only a number."

When you do weigh yourself, it's best to do so at the same time of day, with the same amount of clothing on each time. Shanisha B. weighs herself twice a month now, but did it weekly when she was losing. "If my weight is up," she says, "I don't get upset. I just try to figure out why." (Most experts I talked with suggest that teens in their programs weigh in once a week.)

As you look back over the week, use "I'd like to work on this" to think about your future goals. "Reminders of why I want to get to a healthier weight" allows you to focus on your reasons for wanting to lose weight in the first place. In "Reminders of how my life is better already," you can note the positive changes that are going on in your life — another technique the teens use to stay motivated.

Sandra D. suggests, "Notice that you can do more things — like being less tired after you take part in a fitness test." Other teens talked about having better relationships and more confidence. Tyler D. says, "Look at what you've accomplished and take note of how much healthier, not just thinner, you are compared with before."

In Mary N.'s words, "I think of where I was and how far I've come."

Make this journal your friend. Anytime you feel discouraged, thumb through your weekly review pages to refresh your memory about all the things you've accomplished since you started on your path to a healthier weight.

> "Once you see what it's like, you never, ever want to go back."
> — Aaron T.

Believe you can succeed.

> "Deep down, you really have to *want* to lose weight; no one can force you. You have to believe in yourself."
>
> — McKenzie K.

About McKenzie: At her heaviest, McKenzie weighed 135 pounds and was just 4'10" tall. She decided to do something about her weight when she was 13. At 15½, she's slimmed down to 120 and has grown to 5'3½".

Habits before: "I felt I had to clean my plate."

Turning point: "I was sick of my lifestyle and sick of being fatter than all my friends. I'd been invited to a swimming party and didn't want to look fat in my swimsuit."

How she did it: "I worked out more, skated more, cut out the sweets and high-fat foods, and ate healthier. Now I make sure I have at least five fruits and veggies, including at least one salad, each day. I read labels and eat healthier snacks — like an apple and some pretzels with low-fat dip. I try to distract myself from eating by staying out of the kitchen and keeping busy."

How she stays fit: "All year long, I do figure skating at least 2 to 5 times a week for 60 to 75 minutes. In the fall, I also run on my school's cross-country team."

How can you start to believe in yourself?

"It's easy to believe in yourself when you understand more about who you are. Ask yourself who you are and who you want to be. Figure out goals that you have in life, and write them down. Save them to remind yourself of them when you feel down and out. Include some of your weight and fitness goals, but also include goals that are beyond looks and health."

Find a role model: "It helped me to turn to a friend who eats everything you're supposed to. I would just watch what she did and try to follow. Today, she is still a good role model to me. She works out almost every day, and she eats properly. She eats sweets every once in a while."

Think about someone who inspires you — maybe it's a friend, teacher, or parent who eats healthy foods and exercises regularly. Pay attention to what he or she does, and if you feel comfortable, ask for some tips.

try this:

MCKENZIE'S SANDWICH
Between 2 slices of whole-grain bread, place slices of avocado, cucumber, pepper Jack cheese, green pepper, onion, tomato and some lettuce, and spinach leaves.

my goal(s) for this week:

_____
_____
_____

Things that might trip me up:

_____
_____
_____

How I plan to deal with them:

_____
_____
_____

MY PLAN FOR EXERCISE/PHYSICAL ACTIVITY

Type of activity/length of time   **What I actually did**

Sunday:_____   _____

Monday:_____   _____

Tuesday:_____   _____

Wednesday:_____   _____

Thursday:_____   _____

Friday:_____   _____

Saturday:_____   _____

Daily Diary

Date: _____

Foods, beverages & snacks I had today:

	Food or beverage and amount	Hunger	Calories/Other	Feelings/Mood
MORNING				
AFTERNOON				
EVENING				
	DAILY TOTAL			

Exercise/Physical activities:	Plan for tomorrow:

Today's successes/Random thoughts:

Daily Diary

Date: _____

Hunger: 1 = starving
2 = kind of hungry
3 = not hungry

Foods, beverages & snacks I had today:

	Food or beverage and amount	Hunger	Calories/Other	Feelings/Mood
MORNING				
AFTERNOON				
EVENING				
DAILY TOTAL				

Exercise/Physical activities:	Plan for tomorrow:

Today's successes/Random thoughts:

Daily Diary

Date: _____

Hunger: 1 = starving
2 = kind of hungry
3 = not hungry

Foods, beverages & snacks I had today:

	Food or beverage and amount	Hunger	Calories/Other	Feelings/Mood
MORNING				
AFTERNOON				
EVENING				
DAILY TOTAL				

Exercise/Physical activities:

Plan for tomorrow:

Today's successes/Random thoughts:

Daily Diary

Date: _____

Foods, beverages & snacks I had today:

	Food or beverage and amount	Hunger	Calories/Other	Feelings/Mood
MORNING				
AFTERNOON				
EVENING				
	DAILY TOTAL			

Exercise/Physical activities:	Plan for tomorrow:

Today's successes/Random thoughts:

Daily Diary

Date:_____

Hunger: 1 = starving
2 = kind of hungry
3 = not hungry

Foods, beverages & snacks I had today:

Food or beverage and amount	Hunger	Calories/ Other	Feelings/Mood
DAILY TOTAL			

Exercise/Physical activities:

Plan for tomorrow:

Today's successes/Random thoughts:

Daily Diary

Date:_____

Hunger: 1 = starving
2 = kind of hungry
3 = not hungry

Foods, beverages & snacks I had today:

	Food or beverage and amount	Hunger	Calories/Other	Feelings/Mood
MORNING				
AFTERNOON				
EVENING				
DAILY TOTAL				

Exercise/Physical activities:	Plan for tomorrow:

Today's successes/Random thoughts:

Daily Diary

Date: _____

Foods, beverages & snacks I had today:

	Food or beverage and amount	Hunger	Calories/Other	Feelings/Mood
MORNING				
AFTERNOON				
EVENING				
DAILY TOTAL				

Exercise/Physical activities:

Plan for tomorrow:

Today's successes/Random thoughts:

Review of My Week

Things that really helped this week:

_____
_____
_____

Was/Were my goal(s) met?

_____
_____
_____

I'd like to work on this:

_____
_____
_____

Reminders of why I want to get to a healthier weight:

_____
_____
_____

Reminders of how my life is better already:

_____
_____
_____

MY WEIGHT:_____

MY SPACE

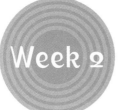

Week 2

Don't let the world get you down.

"Some of my peers made fun of me because of my weight. If they do that to you, use it to motivate yourself."

— Erin D.

About Erin: The most Erin ever weighed was 172, when she was 5'3". At 16, she started on the road to losing 47 pounds. She's now 18, weighs 125 pounds, and is 5'4".

Habits before: She ate for emotional reasons, when she was sad or upset. Her portion sizes were three times larger than they are now.

Turning point: "I started to hate looking in the mirror. I wanted more confidence, didn't like not being able to wear fashionable clothes, and wanted to run faster."

How she did it: "I went on a low-fat, low-calorie diet and snacked on all the fruits and veggies that I wanted. I also ran and did Pilates." Now Erin eats only when she's hungry. "When I go to fast-food restaurants, I'm satisfied with a kid's meal." If she feels like eating for emotional reasons, she writes in her journal or talks to her mom.

How she stays fit: "I run 5 days a week, do Pilates 3 times a week, and do ballet 3 days a week."

How can **you** avoid letting the world get you down?

Jenni O.: "When kids made fun of me I reminded myself that I was beautiful on the inside, and that's what mattered to me."

Emily B.: "Talk to your friends. They can always make you feel better. More often than not, your friends have been teased about something before too, and they know how it feels."

Make a list of things you're good at or accomplishments you're really proud of — tell yourself, "If I can succeed at this, I can also reach a healthier weight."

_____
_____
_____
_____
_____
_____

try this:

ZACH G.'S PITA PIZZA
Preheat the oven to 350°F. Split a small whole-wheat pita in half and toast it. On each half, spread 1 to 2 Tbsp. spaghetti sauce. Place on a cookie sheet or piece of foil. Sprinkle with shredded part-skim mozzarella cheese, plus any chopped veggies you like. Bake for 3 to 5 minutes, until the cheese melts.

my goal(s) for this week:

_____
_____
_____

Things that might trip me up:

_____
_____
_____

How I plan to deal with them:

_____
_____
_____

MY PLAN FOR EXERCISE/PHYSICAL ACTIVITY

Type of activity/length of time

What I actually did

Sunday:_____   _____

Monday:_____   _____

Tuesday:_____   _____

Wednesday:_____   _____

Thursday:_____   _____

Friday:_____   _____

Saturday:_____   _____

Daily Diary

Date: _____

Hunger: 1 = starving
2 = kind of hungry
3 = not hungry

Foods, beverages & snacks I had today:

Food or beverage and amount	Hunger	Calories/Other	Feelings/Mood
DAILY TOTAL			

MORNING

AFTERNOON

EVENING

Exercise/Physical activities:

Plan for tomorrow:

Today's successes/Random thoughts:

Daily Diary

Date: _____

Hunger: 1 = starving
2 = kind of hungry
3 = not hungry

Foods, beverages & snacks I had today:

	Food or beverage and amount	Hunger	Calories/Other	Feelings/Mood
MORNING				
AFTERNOON				
EVENING				
DAILY TOTAL				

Exercise/Physical activities:	Plan for tomorrow:

Today's successes/Random thoughts:

Daily Diary

Date: _____

Foods, beverages & snacks I had today:

	Food or beverage and amount	Hunger	Calories/Other	Feelings/Mood
MORNING				
AFTERNOON				
EVENING				
DAILY TOTAL				

Exercise/Physical activities:

Plan for tomorrow:

Today's successes/Random thoughts:

Daily Diary

Date: _____

Foods, beverages & snacks I had today:

	Food or beverage and amount	Hunger	Calories/ Other	Feelings/Mood
MORNING				
AFTERNOON				
EVENING				
DAILY TOTAL				

Exercise/Physical activities:

Plan for tomorrow:

Today's successes/Random thoughts:

Daily Diary

Date:_____

Foods, beverages & snacks I had today:

Food or beverage and amount	Hunger	Calories/ Other	Feelings/Mood
MORNING			
AFTERNOON			
EVENING			
DAILY TOTAL			

Exercise/Physical activities:

Plan for tomorrow:

Today's successes/Random thoughts:

Daily Diary

Date: _____

Hunger: 1 = starving
2 = kind of hungry
3 = not hungry

Foods, beverages & snacks I had today:

	Food or beverage and amount	Hunger	Calories/Other	Feelings/Mood
MORNING				
AFTERNOON				
EVENING				
DAILY TOTAL				

Exercise/Physical activities:	Plan for tomorrow:

Today's successes/Random thoughts:

Daily Diary

Date:_____

Hunger: 1 = starving

2 = kind of hungry

3 = not hungry

Foods, beverages & snacks I had today:

	Food or beverage and amount	Hunger	Calories/Other	Feelings/Mood
MORNING				
AFTERNOON				
EVENING				
DAILY TOTAL				

Exercise/Physical activities:	Plan for tomorrow:

Today's successes/Random thoughts:

Review of My Week

Things that really helped this week:

_____

_____

_____

Was/Were my goal(s) met?

_____

_____

_____

I'd like to work on this:

_____

_____

_____

Reminders of why I want to get to a healthier weight:

_____

_____

_____

Reminders of how my life is better already:

_____

_____

_____

MY WEIGHT:_____

MY SPACE

Find the right reasons to slim down.

> "It took years for me to find the inspiration, but when I finally got it, there was no stopping me. It's hard to get the ball rolling, but once you do, it's that much harder to stop it."
> — Aaron T.

About Aaron: At 16, he weighed 235 and was 5'9" tall. A year later, he weighs 185 and has grown half an inch.

Habits before: "My biggest problem was large portion sizes."

Turning point: "I wanted to prove to myself I could do anything I set my mind to. The other thing that did it was girls." Aaron also wanted to be fit, like his in-shape dad.

How he did it: Aaron worked with a registered dietician, who helped him follow a healthy diet. "I began thinking about what would fill me up and what was worth it." He also used an elliptical machine, lifted some weights, and ran around a track when time permitted. He now eats more whole grains, drinks more milk and water, and chooses healthier snacks.

How he stays fit: Aaron's exercise varies, depending on how busy he is and the time of year. He does weightlifting, jogging, and sit-ups, and he sometimes uses an elliptical machine for about an hour. "Running a mile for school fitness tests used to be a disaster." Now he can run a 5k race and beat his super-fit dad.

How can you find the right reasons to slim down?

"Unless you want to do something about your weight for good reasons, you probably won't stick with it. If you're happy with the way you look or not unhappy enough to do something about it, then let it be. You'll only feel worse about yourself afterward if you don't succeed." — Sari M.

try this:

WES G.'S PEANUT BUTTER–BANANA ROLL-UP
Spread a whole-wheat tortilla with a light coating of reduced-fat peanut butter. Place a layer of thin banana slices on top of the peanut butter, then roll up the whole thing. (If the tortilla isn't very flexible, zap it in the microwave for 15 to 25 seconds before topping it with the peanut butter.)

Make a list of your reasons for wanting to get to a healthier weight — think not only about how you want to look but also about how you'd like to feel about yourself, your health, your relationships. Think about things you'd like to accomplish. Pull out your list whenever you need some motivation.

_____
_____
_____
_____
_____
_____
_____

my goal(s) for this week:

_____
_____
_____

Things that might trip me up:

_____
_____
_____

How I plan to deal with them:

_____
_____
_____

MY PLAN FOR EXERCISE/PHYSICAL ACTIVITY

Type of activity/length of time   What I actually did

Sunday:_____   _____

Monday:_____   _____

Tuesday:_____   _____

Wednesday:_____   _____

Thursday:_____   _____

Friday:_____   _____

Saturday:_____   _____

Daily Diary

Date: _____

Hunger: 1 = starving
2 = kind of hungry
3 = not hungry

Foods, beverages & snacks I had today:

	Food or beverage and amount	Hunger	Calories/ Other	Feelings/Mood
MORNING				
AFTERNOON				
EVENING				
DAILY TOTAL				

Exercise/Physical activities:	Plan for tomorrow:

Today's successes/Random thoughts:

Daily Diary

Date: _____

Foods, beverages & snacks I had today:

	Food or beverage and amount	Hunger	Calories/ Other	Feelings/Mood
MORNING				
AFTERNOON				
EVENING				
DAILY TOTAL				

Exercise/Physical activities:

Plan for tomorrow:

Today's successes/Random thoughts:

Daily Diary

Date: _____

Hunger: 1 = starving
2 = kind of hungry
3 = not hungry

Foods, beverages & snacks I had today:

	Food or beverage and amount	Hunger	Calories/Other	Feelings/Mood
MORNING				
AFTERNOON				
EVENING				
DAILY TOTAL				

Exercise/Physical activities:	Plan for tomorrow:

Today's successes/Random thoughts:

Daily Diary

Date: _____

Foods, beverages & snacks I had today:

	Food or beverage and amount	Hunger	Calories/Other	Feelings/Mood
MORNING				
AFTERNOON				
EVENING				
DAILY TOTAL				

Exercise/Physical activities:	Plan for tomorrow:

Today's successes/Random thoughts:

Daily Diary

Date: _____

Hunger: 1 = starving
2 = kind of hungry
3 = not hungry

Foods, beverages & snacks I had today:

Food or beverage and amount	Hunger	Calories/Other	Feelings/Mood
MORNING			
AFTERNOON			
EVENING			
DAILY TOTAL			

Exercise/Physical activities:	Plan for tomorrow:

Today's successes/Random thoughts:

Daily Diary

Date: _____

Foods, beverages & snacks I had today:

	Food or beverage and amount	Hunger	Calories/Other	Feelings/Mood
MORNING				
AFTERNOON				
EVENING				
DAILY TOTAL				

Exercise/Physical activities:

Plan for tomorrow:

Today's successes/Random thoughts:

Daily Diary

Date: _____

Hunger: 1 = starving
2 = kind of hungry
3 = not hungry

Foods, beverages & snacks I had today:

	Food or beverage and amount	Hunger	Calories/Other	Feelings/Mood
MORNING				
AFTERNOON				
EVENING				
DAILY TOTAL				

Exercise/Physical activities:	Plan for tomorrow:

Today's successes/Random thoughts:

Review of My Week

Things that really helped this week:

_____
_____
_____

Was/Were my goal(s) met?

_____
_____
_____

I'd like to work on this:

_____
_____
_____

Reminders of why I want to get to a healthier weight:

_____
_____
_____

Reminders of how my life is better already:

_____
_____
_____

MY WEIGHT:_____

MY SPACE

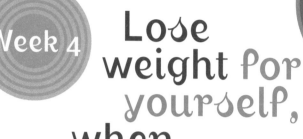

Week 4

Lose weight for yourself, when you're ready.

"I wanted to lose weight for me. My advice to other teens is, 'Do it for yourself.' "

— **Missy S.**

About Missy: Missy's heaviest weight was 240 pounds, when she was 5'5" tall. She decided to slim down when she was 16½. At 18, she weighs 190, and she's grown to 5'9".

Habits before: "I spent too much time in front of the TV and computer and playing video games."

Turning point: "I was sick of people's response to me — they never wanted to get to know me. I know what I am on the inside and wanted them to be able to see that."

How she did it: "I went to the Committed to Kids weight program [now called Trim Kids]. I biked, ran, and did exercise videos. I stopped eating sweets, counted calories, and cut back on fat." She drinks more water and has less soda and fruit drinks. Her treats are fruits, because "they're good substitutes for sweets." When she goes to parties, she has a small piece of cake.

How she stays fit: "I am in the marching band at school, run 2 days a week for 30 minutes, do some biking, and use an exercise video about once a week."

How can you start to lose weight for you?

Athlete Bill S. says he lost 100 pounds partly to please his coaches. But ultimately, he says, "I had to want to do it. I didn't want to go through high school and not be known for anything. I chose to lose weight so I could become a good athlete."

try this:

JORGEY W.'S TOMATO SOUP
Make tomato soup according to the directions on the can. Add some cooked peas and top with a sprinkling of grated Parmesan cheese and some low-fat or fat-free croutons.

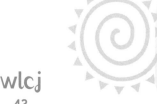

Here are some other questions you can ask yourself to see whether you're ready. The more answers you have on the left-hand side of the scales — in the "very" area — the more likely you are to be ready to take the steps toward reaching a healthier weight.

How much do I want to do something about my weight right now?

Very much ___   Sort of ___   Not much ___

How confident am I that I can do something about my weight?

Very confident ___   Sort of confident ___   Not confident ___

How ready am I to change my eating habits?

Very ready ___   Sort of ready ___   Not ready ___

How ready am I to become more physically active?

Very ready ___   Sort of ready ___   Not ready ___

my goal(s) for this week:

_____

_____

_____

Things that might trip me up: How I plan to deal with them:

_____   _____

_____   _____

_____   _____

MY PLAN FOR EXERCISE/PHYSICAL ACTIVITY

Type of activity/length of time   What I actually did

Sunday: _____   _____

Monday: _____   _____

Tuesday: _____   _____

Wednesday: _____   _____

Thursday: _____   _____

Friday: _____   _____

Saturday: _____   _____

Daily Diary

Date: _____

Foods, beverages & snacks I had today:

	Food or beverage and amount	Hunger	Calories/Other	Feelings/Mood
MORNING				
AFTERNOON				
EVENING				
DAILY TOTAL				

Exercise/Physical activities:

Plan for tomorrow:

Today's successes/Random thoughts:

Daily Diary

Date: _____

Hunger: 1 = starving
2 = kind of hungry
3 = not hungry

Foods, beverages & snacks I had today:

	Food or beverage and amount	Hunger	Calories/Other	Feelings/Mood
MORNING				
AFTERNOON				
EVENING				
DAILY TOTAL				

Exercise/Physical activities:

Plan for tomorrow:

Today's successes/Random thoughts:

Daily Diary

Date: _____

Hunger: 1 = starving
2 = kind of hungry
3 = not hungry

Foods, beverages & snacks I had today:

	Food or beverage and amount	Hunger	Calories/ Other	Feelings/Mood
MORNING				
AFTERNOON				
EVENING				
DAILY TOTAL				

Exercise/Physical activities:

Plan for tomorrow:

Today's successes/Random thoughts:

Daily Diary

Date: _____

Foods, beverages & snacks I had today:

	Food or beverage and amount	Hunger	Calories/Other	Feelings/Mood
MORNING				
AFTERNOON				
EVENING				
DAILY TOTAL				

Exercise/Physical activities:	Plan for tomorrow:

Today's successes/Random thoughts:

Daily Diary

Date:_____

Foods, beverages & snacks I had today:

	Food or beverage and amount	Hunger	Calories/Other	Feelings/Mood
MORNING				
AFTERNOON				
EVENING				
DAILY TOTAL				

Exercise/Physical activities:	Plan for tomorrow:

Today's successes/Random thoughts:

Daily Diary

Date:_____

Hunger: 1 = starving
2 = kind of hungry
3 = not hungry

Foods, beverages & snacks I had today:

	Food or beverage and amount	Hunger	Calories/ Other	Feelings/Mood
MORNING				
AFTERNOON				
EVENING				
DAILY TOTAL				

Exercise/Physical activities:	Plan for tomorrow:

Today's successes/Random thoughts:

week 4 — day 6   49

Daily Diary

Date: _____

Foods, beverages & snacks I had today:

	Food or beverage and amount	Hunger	Calories/Other	Feelings/Mood
MORNING				
AFTERNOON				
EVENING				
DAILY TOTAL				

Exercise/Physical activities:

Plan for tomorrow:

Today's successes/Random thoughts:

Review of My Week

Things that really helped this week:

_____
_____
_____

Was/Were my goal(s) met?

_____
_____
_____

I'd like to work on this:

_____
_____
_____

Reminders of why I want to get to a healthier weight:

_____
_____
_____

Reminders of how my life is better already:

_____
_____
_____

MY WEIGHT:_____

MY SPACE

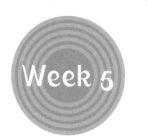

Don't Fall into Fad diets.

> "I got tangled up in two crazy fad diets before I took my own approach. I managed to lose about 10 pounds but piled it back on. Then I ended up getting really sick and missing school."
>
> — Jeana S.

About Jeana: In the 8th grade, Jeana weighed 152 pounds. During high school, she got down to 140, then she lost another 10 pounds as a college student. She's 22 and has weighed 130 for about 2 years. (She is 5'3".)

Habits before: "A lot of little things added up — I started doing more schoolwork and did less work around my parents' dairy farm. I'd eat huge bowlfuls of cereal at midnight and ate a lot socially with friends."

Turning point: "I'd vowed I'd never top 150 pounds. When I hit 152, I knew it was time to do something." After the fad diets failed, Jeana visited relatives who got her hooked on walking and good-tasting, healthy foods. "It was then that I made the connection that eating and exercising have to go hand in hand."

How she did it: "I focused on eating healthy foods, ate 6 mini-meals a day, packed my own lunch, and followed the Food Guide Pyramid." Jeana still eats healthy foods such as fruits, vegetables, beans, and whole grains. And she avoids "foods with empty calories" such as sugary products.

How she stays fit: "I do a variety of activities — like lift weights, walk, run, swim, or bike — and aim for 60 minutes of moderate intensity 6 times a week."

try this:

AARON T.'S BLACK BEANS AND RICE

Dice 2 medium onions and mince 2 garlic cloves. Sauté them in a little olive oil in a large nonstick pan over medium-high heat until softened. Stir in 2 chopped bell peppers (red, yellow, or orange), 2 cans drained black beans, a 28-oz. can diced tomatoes, $1^1/_2$ tsp. cumin powder, 1 tsp. chili powder, and some black pepper and crushed red pepper flakes, to suit your taste. Turn the heat to low, cover, and cook for about 45 minutes, stirring occasionally. Spoon over white or brown rice and sprinkle with some reduced-fat or nonfat cheddar cheese.

wlcj

What healthy strategies do you want to concentrate on?

To get to a healthier weight, the teens used these strategies:

- Exercised more
- Went to a weight-loss program or got help from a professional
- Cut back on foods high in fat
- Went on a healthy diet
- Stopped eating certain foods
- Counted calories
- Ate all foods, just less of them

Which ones are you willing to try?

_____

_____

_____

_____

my goal(s) for this week:

_____

_____

_____

Things that might trip me up:	How I plan to deal with them:
_____	_____
_____	_____
_____	_____

MY PLAN FOR EXERCISE/PHYSICAL ACTIVITY

Type of activity/length of time	What I actually did
Sunday:_____	_____
Monday:_____	_____
Tuesday:_____	_____
Wednesday:_____	_____
Thursday:_____	_____
Friday:_____	_____
Saturday:_____	_____

Daily Diary

Date:_____

Foods, beverages & snacks I had today:

	Food or beverage and amount	Hunger	Calories/Other	Feelings/Mood
MORNING				
AFTERNOON				
EVENING				
DAILY TOTAL				

Exercise/Physical activities:

Plan for tomorrow:

Today's successes/Random thoughts:

Daily Diary

Date:_____

Foods, beverages & snacks I had today:

	Food or beverage and amount	Hunger	Calories/Other	Feelings/Mood
MORNING				
AFTERNOON				
EVENING				
DAILY TOTAL				

Exercise/Physical activities:	Plan for tomorrow:

Today's successes/Random thoughts:

Daily Diary

Date:_____

Foods, beverages & snacks I had today:

	Food or beverage and amount	Hunger	Calories/Other	Feelings/Mood
MORNING				
AFTERNOON				
EVENING				
DAILY TOTAL				

Exercise/Physical activities:

Plan for tomorrow:

Today's successes/Random thoughts:

Daily Diary

Date: _____

Hunger: 1 = starving
2 = kind of hungry
3 = not hungry

Foods, beverages & snacks I had today:

	Food or beverage and amount	Hunger	Calories/Other	Feelings/Mood
MORNING				
AFTERNOON				
EVENING				
DAILY TOTAL				

Exercise/Physical activities:	Plan for tomorrow:

Today's successes/Random thoughts:

Daily Diary

Date: _____

Hunger: 1 = starving
          2 = kind of hungry
          3 = not hungry

Foods, beverages & snacks I had today:

	Food or beverage and amount	Hunger	Calories/ Other	Feelings/Mood
MORNING				
AFTERNOON				
EVENING				
DAILY TOTAL				

Exercise/Physical activities:	Plan for tomorrow:

Today's successes/Random thoughts:

Daily Diary

Date:_____

Hunger: 1 = starving
2 = kind of hungry
3 = not hungry

Foods, beverages & snacks I had today:

	Food or beverage and amount	Hunger	Calories/ Other	Feelings/Mood
MORNING				
AFTERNOON				
EVENING				
DAILY TOTAL				

Exercise/Physical activities:	Plan for tomorrow:

Today's successes/Random thoughts:

Daily Diary

Date:_____

Hunger: 1 = starving
2 = kind of hungry
3 = not hungry

Foods, beverages & snacks I had today:

	Food or beverage and amount	Hunger	Calories/Other	Feelings/Mood
MORNING				
AFTERNOON				
EVENING				
DAILY TOTAL				

Exercise/Physical activities:	Plan for tomorrow:

Today's successes/Random thoughts:

Review of My Week

Things that really helped this week:

_____
_____
_____

Was/Were my goal(s) met?

_____
_____
_____

I'd like to work on this:

_____
_____
_____

Reminders of why I want to get to a healthier weight:

_____
_____
_____

Reminders of how my life is better already:

_____
_____
_____

MY WEIGHT:_____

MY SPACE

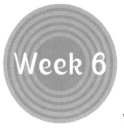

Get around what's getting in the way of exercising.

About Marie: Marie's highest weight was 175 pounds. At 17, she started slimming down to her current weight of 120. She's now 22½, and her height remains at 5'4".

Habits before: "I used to eat anything and everything I could get my hands on, regardless of my hunger level."

Turning point: "I wanted to take control of the way I was eating and to be better at sports."

"Exercise increased my energy level and helped me feel better about myself. Just get moving — and make sure you have fun."

— Marie P.

How she did it: "I joined school teams—ice hockey, field hockey, softball—and started working out on my own. With my mother's help, I watched what and how often I ate and learned as much as I could about healthy eating." She now focuses on healthy foods, like fruits, vegetables, and whole grains, and "listens" to her hunger. "In moderation," she allows herself a daily treat.

How she stays fit: "I run 4 days a week for 35 minutes and do strength training 3 or 4 days a week for 15 minutes."

How can you get around what's getting in the way of exercising?

Mick J.: "When I was overweight, I was too self-conscious to exercise in public. So my mom bought a treadmill, and I was able to start exercising in the privacy of my own home."

Sandra D.: "If you're uncomfortable working out with bodybuilding men, then look for a gym more tailored to your interests, such as an all-women's gym."

What's getting in your way with exercise, and how can you get around the obstacles?

_____
_____
_____
_____
_____
_____

my goal(s) for this week:

_____
_____
_____

Things that might trip me up:	How I plan to deal with them:
_____	_____
_____	_____
_____	_____

MY PLAN FOR EXERCISE/PHYSICAL ACTIVITY

Type of activity/length of time	What I actually did
Sunday:_____	_____
Monday:_____	_____
Tuesday:_____	_____
Wednesday:_____	_____
Thursday:_____	_____
Friday:_____	_____
Saturday:_____	_____

Daily Diary

Date: _____

Hunger: 1 = starving
2 = kind of hungry
3 = not hungry

Foods, beverages & snacks I had today:

	Food or beverage and amount	Hunger	Calories/Other	Feelings/Mood
MORNING				
AFTERNOON				
EVENING				
DAILY TOTAL				

Exercise/Physical activities:	Plan for tomorrow:

Today's successes/Random thoughts:

Daily Diary

Date: _____

Foods, beverages & snacks I had today:

	Food or beverage and amount	Hunger	Calories/Other	Feelings/Mood
MORNING				
AFTERNOON				
EVENING				
DAILY TOTAL				

Exercise/Physical activities:	Plan for tomorrow:

Today's successes/Random thoughts:

Daily Diary

Date: _____

Foods, beverages & snacks I had today:

	Food or beverage and amount	Hunger	Calories/ Other	Feelings/Mood
MORNING				
AFTERNOON				
EVENING				
DAILY TOTAL				

Exercise/Physical activities:	Plan for tomorrow:

Today's successes/Random thoughts:

Daily Diary

Date:_____

Hunger: 1 = starving
2 = kind of hungry
3 = not hungry

Foods, beverages & snacks I had today:

	Food or beverage and amount	Hunger	Calories/Other	Feelings/Mood
MORNING				
AFTERNOON				
EVENING				
DAILY TOTAL				

Exercise/Physical activities:	Plan for tomorrow:

Today's successes/Random thoughts:

week 6 — day 4   67

Daily Diary

Date:_____

Hunger: 1 = starving
        2 = kind of hungry
        3 = not hungry

Foods, beverages & snacks I had today:

	Food or beverage and amount	Hunger	Calories/Other	Feelings/Mood
MORNING				
AFTERNOON				
EVENING				
DAILY TOTAL				

Exercise/Physical activities:

Plan for tomorrow:

Today's successes/Random thoughts:

Daily Diary

Date: _____

Foods, beverages & snacks I had today:

Food or beverage and amount	Hunger	Calories/Other	Feelings/Mood
MORNING			
AFTERNOON			
EVENING			
DAILY TOTAL			

Exercise/Physical activities:	Plan for tomorrow:

Today's successes/Random thoughts:

Daily Diary

Date:_____

Hunger: 1 = starving
2 = kind of hungry
3 = not hungry

Foods, beverages & snacks I had today:

	Food or beverage and amount	Hunger	Calories/Other	Feelings/Mood
MORNING				
AFTERNOON				
EVENING				
DAILY TOTAL				

Exercise/Physical activities:	Plan for tomorrow:

Today's successes/Random thoughts:

Review of My Week

Things that really helped this week:

_____

_____

_____

Was/Were my goal(s) met?

_____

_____

_____

I'd like to work on this:

_____

_____

_____

Reminders of why I want to get to a healthier weight:

_____

_____

_____

Reminders of how my life is better already:

_____

_____

_____

MY WEIGHT:_____

MY SPACE

Eat regular meals.

> "I never used to eat anything for breakfast, but then I read a study that said eating nothing is really bad for you. Needless to say, I have breakfast now."
>
> — Tyler D.

About Tyler: Tyler D. began gaining too much weight when he was 9, after his doctor placed him on powerful medications for his severe asthma. At the age of 13, he weighed 185 pounds and was 5'4" tall. At 14, he started slimming down. Today he's a slender 20-year-old college student who weighs 165 pounds and is 6'1".

Habits before: Irregular meals and too much snacking. Because of asthma attacks, Ty didn't exercise much.

Turning point: When he got to the 7th grade, Tyler got sick of being overweight and being teased and "just made up his mind" that he wasn't going to gain another pound.

How he did it: Ty went from "eating whenever I wanted" to eating 3 times a day, "breakfast, lunch, and dinner." He stopped nighttime snacking and drank more water. Gradually, he became an athlete. He joined the middle school football team and was told he was too heavy for the position he wanted to play. Still, Ty stuck with the team and kept his vow not to gain any more weight. Later that school year, he went out for track and made the team. He slimmed down gradually and advanced slowly but surely to varsity football, then became one of the front-runners on a track team that won second place in the state championship his senior year.

How he stays fit: Ty's exercise varies with the season — on average, he does something 5 days a week for an hour. His activities include running, biking, playing basketball or catch football with friends, and lifting weights.

How can you eat regular meals?

Nearly three quarters of the teens said that they regularly eat breakfast, a morning snack, or both. And 9 out of 10 of them eat lunch. In fact, the vast majority of the teens eat breakfast, lunch, and dinner.

What meals do you usually skip?

_____

_____

_____

List foods for 3 easy, healthy breakfasts or lunches you're willing to try.

_____

_____

_____

my goal(s) for this week:

_____

_____

_____

Things that might trip me up:

_____

_____

_____

How I plan to deal with them:

_____

_____

_____

MY PLAN FOR EXERCISE/PHYSICAL ACTIVITY

Type of activity/length of time   What I actually did

Sunday:_____   _____

Monday:_____   _____

Tuesday:_____   _____

Wednesday:_____   _____

Thursday:_____   _____

Friday:_____   _____

Saturday:_____   _____

Daily Diary

Date: _____

Hunger: 1 = starving
2 = kind of hungry
3 = not hungry

Foods, beverages & snacks I had today:

	Food or beverage and amount	Hunger	Calories/Other	Feelings/Mood
MORNING				
AFTERNOON				
EVENING				
DAILY TOTAL				

Exercise/Physical activities:	Plan for tomorrow:

Today's successes/Random thoughts:

Daily Diary

Date: _____

Hunger: 1 = starving
2 = kind of hungry
3 = not hungry

Foods, beverages & snacks I had today:

	Food or beverage and amount	Hunger	Calories/Other	Feelings/Mood
MORNING				
AFTERNOON				
EVENING				
	DAILY TOTAL			

Exercise/Physical activities:	Plan for tomorrow:
Today's successes/Random thoughts:	

Daily Diary

Date: _____

Hunger: 1 = starving
           2 = kind of hungry
           3 = not hungry

Foods, beverages & snacks I had today:

	Food or beverage and amount	Hunger	Calories/Other	Feelings/Mood
MORNING				
AFTERNOON				
EVENING				
DAILY TOTAL				

Exercise/Physical activities:

Plan for tomorrow:

Today's successes/Random thoughts:

Daily Diary

Date:_____

Hunger: 1 = starving
2 = kind of hungry
3 = not hungry

Foods, beverages & snacks I had today:

	Food or beverage and amount	Hunger	Calories/Other	Feelings/Mood
MORNING				
AFTERNOON				
EVENING				
DAILY TOTAL				

Exercise/Physical activities:	Plan for tomorrow:

Today's successes/Random thoughts:

Daily Diary

Date:_____

Foods, beverages & snacks I had today:

	Food or beverage and amount	Hunger	Calories/ Other	Feelings/Mood
MORNING				
AFTERNOON				
EVENING				
DAILY TOTAL				

Exercise/Physical activities:	Plan for tomorrow:

Today's successes/Random thoughts:

Daily Diary

Date: _____

Foods, beverages & snacks I had today:

	Food or beverage and amount	Hunger	Calories/ Other	Feelings/Mood
MORNING				
AFTERNOON				
EVENING				
	DAILY TOTAL			

Exercise/Physical activities:	Plan for tomorrow:

Today's successes/Random thoughts:

Daily Diary

Date: _____

Hunger: 1 = starving
2 = kind of hungry
3 = not hungry

Foods, beverages & snacks I had today:

	Food or beverage and amount	Hunger	Calories/Other	Feelings/Mood
MORNING				
AFTERNOON				
EVENING				
DAILY TOTAL				

Exercise/Physical activities:

Plan for tomorrow:

Today's successes/Random thoughts:

80   week 7 — day 7

Review of My Week

Things that really helped this week:

_____

_____

_____

Was/Were my goal(s) met?

_____

_____

_____

I'd like to work on this:

_____

_____

_____

Reminders of why I want to get to a healthier weight:

_____

_____

_____

Reminders of how my life is better already:

_____

_____

_____

MY WEIGHT:_____

MY SPACE

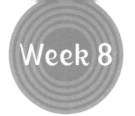

Week 8

Change what you drink.

> "My parents used to try to get me to drink Diet Coke. But that was like admitting I was fat, so I'd sneak regular. Now I won't drink anything *but* Diet Coke. I drink a lot of bottled water too. I stay away from sports drinks, because most are just sugar with some nutrients added."
>
> — Sid J.

About Sid: Sid's weight had climbed to 183 pounds by the time he was 14 (he was 5'3"), which made him a target of teasing. His two older brothers were not overweight, and one of them ate a lot without gaining weight because he was an athlete. At 14½, Sid began slimming down to his current weight of 141— he's 5'7" and 17 years old now.

Habits before: "I had no limits. I ate till I got full and kept eating. When I had fast food, I'd eat all the fries and want more. I'd eat all day and have seconds on desserts."

Turning point: Toward the end of 8th grade, Sid's mother asked whether he'd be willing to go to the first meeting of a new kids' weight program at their local hospital. He agreed: his bar mitzvah was coming up, and he wanted to look good.

How he did it: Sid signed up for the Way to Go Kids! nutrition and fitness program, developed by two registered dietitians. Within the first month, he went from 183 to 170. "It all started working, so I kept going. I just continued doing what I learned in class, and I'm still doing it 3 years later." The program's overall message is, "You shouldn't deprive yourself — eat things in moderation." In addition, Sid took karate lessons and regularly walked on his family's treadmill. He pays attention to food labels and portion sizes, eats healthier snacks, and tries not to eat too much fat or sugar.

How he stays fit: Sid does weightlifting and calisthenics at home, about 5 times a week.

try this:

WES G.'S BREAKFAST SHAKE

In a blender, place 1 c. nonfat milk, 1 tsp. vanilla extract, and 1 frozen banana broken into 1- to 2-in. sections. (If you want, add a packet of no-calorie sweetener.) Blend until smooth. (When bananas are starting to become overripe, put them in a plastic bag, close it, then flatten them and freeze. They'll break easily that way.)

How can you change what you drink?

- ➤ "I drink water instead of juice or soda. I'd rather use my calories on food items instead of drinking them." — Bella S.
- ➤ Switch to diet soda.
- ➤ "Get yourself a water bottle and carry it with you everywhere." — Jeana S.
- ➤ "Try flavored water if plain gets too boring." — McKenzie K.
- ➤ "One of my favorite things is Crystal Light packets that you can throw into a 20-oz. bottle of water and shake up." — Erin D.
- ➤ When you have milk, stick with fat-free.

What's your plan for changing what you drink?

_____

my goal(s) for this week:

_____
_____
_____

Things that might trip me up:	How I plan to deal with them:
_____	_____
_____	_____
_____	_____

MY PLAN FOR EXERCISE/PHYSICAL ACTIVITY

Type of activity/length of time	What I actually did
Sunday:	
Monday:	
Tuesday:	
Wednesday:	
Thursday:	
Friday:	
Saturday:	

Daily Diary

Date: _____

Hunger: 1 = starving
2 = kind of hungry
3 = not hungry

Foods, beverages & snacks I had today:

	Food or beverage and amount	Hunger	Calories/Other	Feelings/Mood
MORNING				
AFTERNOON				
EVENING				
DAILY TOTAL				

Exercise/Physical activities:	Plan for tomorrow:

Today's successes/Random thoughts:

Daily Diary

Date:_____

Hunger: 1 = starving
2 = kind of hungry
3 = not hungry

Foods, beverages & snacks I had today:

	Food or beverage and amount	Hunger	Calories/ Other	Feelings/Mood
MORNING				
AFTERNOON				
EVENING				
DAILY TOTAL				

Exercise/Physical activities:	Plan for tomorrow:

Today's successes/Random thoughts:

Daily Diary

Date: _____

Hunger: 1 = starving
2 = kind of hungry
3 = not hungry

Foods, beverages & snacks I had today:

	Food or beverage and amount	Hunger	Calories/ Other	Feelings/Mood
MORNING				
AFTERNOON				
EVENING				
DAILY TOTAL				

Exercise/Physical activities:	Plan for tomorrow:

Today's successes/Random thoughts:

Daily Diary

Date: _____

Hunger: 1 = starving
        2 = kind of hungry
        3 = not hungry

Foods, beverages & snacks I had today:

	Food or beverage and amount	Hunger	Calories/Other	Feelings/Mood
MORNING				
AFTERNOON				
EVENING				
DAILY TOTAL				

Exercise/Physical activities:

Plan for tomorrow:

Today's successes/Random thoughts:

Daily Diary

Date: _____

Hunger: 1 = starving
2 = kind of hungry
3 = not hungry

Foods, beverages & snacks I had today:

	Food or beverage and amount	Hunger	Calories/Other	Feelings/Mood
MORNING				
AFTERNOON				
EVENING				
DAILY TOTAL				

Exercise/Physical activities:	Plan for tomorrow:

Today's successes/Random thoughts:

Daily Diary

Date: _____

Hunger: 1 = starving
2 = kind of hungry
3 = not hungry

Foods, beverages & snacks I had today:

	Food or beverage and amount	Hunger	Calories/Other	Feelings/Mood
MORNING				
AFTERNOON				
EVENING				
DAILY TOTAL				

Exercise/Physical activities:	Plan for tomorrow:

Today's successes/Random thoughts:

Daily Diary

Date: _____

Hunger: 1 = starving
2 = kind of hungry
3 = not hungry

Foods, beverages & snacks I had today:

	Food or beverage and amount	Hunger	Calories/Other	Feelings/Mood
MORNING				
AFTERNOON				
EVENING				
DAILY TOTAL				

Exercise/Physical activities:	Plan for tomorrow:

Today's successes/Random thoughts:

Review of My Week

Things that really helped this week:

_____

_____

_____

Was/Were my goal(s) met?

_____

_____

_____

I'd like to work on this:

_____

_____

_____

Reminders of why I want to get to a healthier weight:

_____

_____

_____

Reminders of how my life is better already:

_____

_____

_____

MY WEIGHT:_____

MY SPACE

Let your family know what helps—and what doesn't help.

About Sean: He started losing weight when he was 12½, weighed 170 pounds, and stood 5'3" tall. A college sophomore, Sean is 19, weighs 165 pounds, and is 5'8".

Habits before: "I overate in general."

Turning point: "Girls!" Sean was also sick of being teased and wanted to do better at sports and be healthier.

How he did it: "I asked my parents to buy me a treadmill and followed a low-fat diet. Now I'm constantly aware of what I eat. I avoid fatty, sugary foods and eat more fruits and veggies. I eat a constant, healthy diet and don't go in and out of 'dieting.'" His parents got off his back about what he ate and left the decisions up to him.

How he stays fit: "I lift weights for 40 minutes, 3 or 4 days a week, and play basketball once a week."

"If I came home for dinner and didn't eat much, my parents used to ask, 'What were you eating before dinner?' I'd deny it, and then proceed to feel terrible, which only made me want to eat more. Left to my own devices, I decided it was in my best interest to make the changes."

— Sean C.

How can you let your family know what helps — and what doesn't help?

John W.: "Teenagers need to be talked to like a friend. The last person they want to listen to is a disciplinarian parent laying down the law about 'this is why you need to lose weight.'"

Kyle B.'s advice to parents: "Don't plan a teen's diet for him or her. Let your child learn what works and what doesn't on his own."

Emily B.: "If your teen messes up, don't get angry."

What are some things your family does that are not helpful?

_____

_____

What are some things your family can do to help you manage your weight?
Would you like them to help you find a weight program, stock healthier foods, praise your efforts, buy exercise equipment, or join you losing weight and being more active?

_____

_____

try this:

"Brush your teeth after you eat or when you feel you've had enough. It keeps you from eating more than you should because you can be like, 'I just brushed my teeth and don't want to brush them again.'" — McKenzie K.

my goal(s) for this week:

_____

_____

_____

Things that might trip me up:

_____

_____

_____

How I plan to deal with them:

_____

_____

_____

MY PLAN FOR EXERCISE/PHYSICAL ACTIVITY

Type of activity/length of time

What I actually did

Sunday:_____   _____

Monday:_____   _____

Tuesday:_____   _____

Wednesday:_____   _____

Thursday:_____   _____

Friday:_____   _____

Saturday:_____   _____

Daily Diary

Date: _____

Hunger: 1 = starving
2 = kind of hungry
3 = not hungry

Foods, beverages & snacks I had today:

	Food or beverage and amount	Hunger	Calories/Other	Feelings/Mood
MORNING				
AFTERNOON				
EVENING				
DAILY TOTAL				

Exercise/Physical activities:	Plan for tomorrow:

Today's successes/Random thoughts:

Daily Diary

Date: _____

Foods, beverages & snacks I had today:

	Food or beverage and amount	Hunger	Calories/Other	Feelings/Mood
MORNING				
AFTERNOON				
EVENING				
DAILY TOTAL				

Exercise/Physical activities:	Plan for tomorrow:

Today's successes/Random thoughts:

Daily Diary

Date: _____

Hunger: 1 = starving
2 = kind of hungry
3 = not hungry

Foods, beverages & snacks I had today:

	Food or beverage and amount	Hunger	Calories/Other	Feelings/Mood
MORNING				
AFTERNOON				
EVENING				
DAILY TOTAL				

Exercise/Physical activities:

Plan for tomorrow:

Today's successes/Random thoughts:

Daily Diary

Date: _____

Foods, beverages & snacks I had today:

Food or beverage and amount	Hunger	Calories/ Other	Feelings/Mood
DAILY TOTAL			

(rows grouped as MORNING, AFTERNOON, EVENING)

Exercise/Physical activities:	Plan for tomorrow:

Today's successes/Random thoughts:

Daily Diary

Date: _____

Hunger: 1 = starving
2 = kind of hungry
3 = not hungry

Foods, beverages & snacks I had today:

	Food or beverage and amount	Hunger	Calories/Other	Feelings/Mood
MORNING				
AFTERNOON				
EVENING				
DAILY TOTAL				

Exercise/Physical activities:

Plan for tomorrow:

Today's successes/Random thoughts:

Daily Diary

Date: _____

Foods, beverages & snacks I had today:

Food or beverage and amount	Hunger	Calories/ Other	Feelings/Mood
MORNING			
AFTERNOON			
EVENING			
DAILY TOTAL			

Exercise/Physical activities:	Plan for tomorrow:

Today's successes/Random thoughts:

Daily Diary

Date:_____

Hunger: 1 = starving
2 = kind of hungry
3 = not hungry

Foods, beverages & snacks I had today:

	Food or beverage and amount	Hunger	Calories/Other	Feelings/Mood
MORNING				
AFTERNOON				
EVENING				
DAILY TOTAL				

Exercise/Physical activities:

Plan for tomorrow:

Today's successes/Random thoughts:

Review of My Week

Things that really helped this week:

_____

_____

_____

Was/Were my goal(s) met?

_____

_____

_____

I'd like to work on this:

_____

_____

_____

Reminders of why I want to get to a healthier weight:

_____

_____

_____

Reminders of how my life is better already:

_____

_____

_____

MY WEIGHT:_____

MY SPACE

Downsize portions.

> "I eat anything I want; I just make sure it's portioned appropriately. I eat less of everything than I used to."
>
> — Cassey H.

About Cassey: Cassey's weight maxed out at 285, when he was 5'10" tall. He started slimming down when he was 16. He's 18 and weighs 205 — plus he's grown to 6'2".

Habits before: Big portion sizes were the number one culprit in Cassey's weight gain.

Turning point: "I was always the last to get picked at any athletic game. After a 50-mile hike in the Colorado Rockies with the Boy Scouts, where I was the slowest, I decided I needed to lose weight."

How he did it: Without much success, he tried for several months to lose weight on his own. At the same time, his parents were losing weight by going to weekly meetings of the TOPS (Take Off Pounds Sensibly) program. "When I saw how much weight my mom had lost, I decided it was worth a try." He went to TOPS meetings, exercised regularly, cut back on portion sizes and snacks, and ate less fast food. And he still goes to TOPS meetings twice a month.

How he stays fit: "I lift weights 3 times a week for 30 minutes and bike 3 times a week for 30 minutes."

How can you downsize portions?

Before losing weight, Zach G. says, "I thought the nutrition facts on the label were for the whole bag or package, not for individual portions." (On the label's Nutrition Facts panel, pay careful attention to serving size, then to the number of calories in that size.)

Tara G.: "For my morning cereal, I use a small bowl and fill it to the top. It makes me think I'm getting more."

Sid J. lets the label be his guide to a single portion size — he doesn't eat out of the bag or box.

Molly S.: "Don't put food in serving dishes out on the table. Instead, each person should make his own plate, with no second helpings."

Nicole S. weighs and measures her food. Use these rough portion guides.

1 ounce of hard cheese = 4 dice

1 medium potato = a computer mouse

3 ounces of meat, fish, or poultry = a deck of cards

$1/2$ cup of cooked rice = a cupcake wrapper full

1 cup of cereal or cooked pasta = a fist

What can you do to downsize portions?

_____

_____

try this:

MARY N.'S CHEESECAKE SUBSTITUTE
Mix 1 oz. low-fat or nonfat cream cheese with a packet of Splenda and spread it on a graham cracker.

my goal(s) for this week:

_____

_____

_____

Things that might trip me up:

_____

_____

_____

How I plan to deal with them:

_____

_____

_____

MY PLAN FOR EXERCISE/PHYSICAL ACTIVITY

Type of activity/length of time   **What I actually did**

Sunday:_____   _____

Monday:_____   _____

Tuesday:_____   _____

Wednesday:_____   _____

Thursday:_____   _____

Friday:_____   _____

Saturday:_____   _____

Daily Diary

Date: _____

Foods, beverages & snacks I had today:

	Food or beverage and amount	Hunger	Calories/ Other	Feelings/Mood
MORNING				
AFTERNOON				
EVENING				
DAILY TOTAL				

Exercise/Physical activities:

Plan for tomorrow:

Today's successes/Random thoughts:

Daily Diary

Date:_____

Foods, beverages & snacks I had today:

	Food or beverage and amount	Hunger	Calories/Other	Feelings/Mood
MORNING				
AFTERNOON				
EVENING				
DAILY TOTAL				

Exercise/Physical activities:

Plan for tomorrow:

Today's successes/Random thoughts:

Daily Diary

Date:_____

Hunger: 1 = starving
2 = kind of hungry
3 = not hungry

Foods, beverages & snacks I had today:

Food or beverage and amount	Hunger	Calories/Other	Feelings/Mood

MORNING

AFTERNOON

EVENING

| DAILY TOTAL | | | |

Exercise/Physical activities:

Plan for tomorrow:

Today's successes/Random thoughts:

week 10 — day 3

Daily Diary

Date: _____

Foods, beverages & snacks I had today:

Food or beverage and amount	Hunger	Calories/Other	Feelings/Mood
DAILY TOTAL			

MORNING

AFTERNOON

EVENING

Exercise/Physical activities:	Plan for tomorrow:

Today's successes/Random thoughts:

Daily Diary

Date: _____

Hunger: 1 = starving
2 = kind of hungry
3 = not hungry

Foods, beverages & snacks I had today:

	Food or beverage and amount	Hunger	Calories/ Other	Feelings/Mood
MORNING				
AFTERNOON				
EVENING				
DAILY TOTAL				

Exercise/Physical activities:

Plan for tomorrow:

Today's successes/Random thoughts:

108   week 10 — day 5

Daily Diary

Date: _____

Hunger: 1 = starving
2 = kind of hungry
3 = not hungry

Foods, beverages & snacks I had today:

Food or beverage and amount	Hunger	Calories/Other	Feelings/Mood
MORNING			
AFTERNOON			
EVENING			
DAILY TOTAL			

Exercise/Physical activities:	Plan for tomorrow:

Today's successes/Random thoughts:

Daily Diary

Date:_____

Foods, beverages & snacks I had today:

	Food or beverage and amount	Hunger	Calories/Other	Feelings/Mood
MORNING				
AFTERNOON				
EVENING				
	DAILY TOTAL			

Exercise/Physical activities:	Plan for tomorrow:

Today's successes/Random thoughts:

Review of My Week

Things that really helped this week:

_____
_____
_____

Was/Were my goal(s) met?

_____
_____
_____

I'd like to work on this:

_____
_____
_____

Reminders of why I want to get to a healthier weight:

_____
_____
_____

Reminders of how my life is better already:

_____
_____
_____

MY WEIGHT:_____

MY SPACE

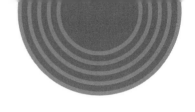

Week 11

Cut the Fat.

> "The most important things I did to lose weight were to stop eating junk food and to avoid being around fatty foods."
>
> — Shanisha B.

About Shanisha: She decided to take charge of her weight at the age of 12, when she weighed 210 pounds and was 5'7" tall. Now 14½, she weighs 170 and is 5'7½".

Habits before: "I wouldn't eat much during the day, then I'd eat a lot at night. I could eat five bags of chips in three minutes."

Turning point: "I couldn't wear what I wanted. And I couldn't do things like run, walk, or play without resting in between. I was going into high school and I wanted to look good."

How she did it: Shanisha went to the FitMatters weight program for children and teens at La Rabida Children's Hospital in Chicago. She followed a low-fat diet and recorded what she ate, along with the fat grams, in a booklet. She measured almost everything she ate using measuring cups and spoons. Shanisha's whole family got involved in planning healthier meals and using healthier recipes. She also went to a gym. She still avoids fatty foods and writes down what she eats about 3 days a week. "When I go to the mall with friends," she says, "I eat at Subway and usually order a sub with turkey or ham and mustard instead of mayonnaise."

How she stays fit: "I walk every day for about an hour or two, run 1 day a week for 20 minutes, and go to the gym 3 times a week."

How can you cut the Fat?

Jack F.: "I avoid all notoriously fatty foods and greasy ways of preparing foods. I only eat fat-free salad dressing, and I never eat mayo. And I never eat at burger fast-food places."

Aaron T.: "I found a great mustard and stuck to it." He also uses hot sauce as a flavoring.

James G.: "I've ruled out fried foods and replaced them with grilled foods."

Lee J.: "Order salad dressing on the side. Dip your fork in the dressing before putting the salad on your fork."

Sid J.: "Something can be fat-free and still be loaded with sugar."

What fatty foods can you cut down on or cut out? Or can you switch to lower-fat versions?

_____
_____
_____
_____

**JORGEY W.'S
LOW-FAT FRIES**
Preheat the oven to 375°F. Spray a cookie sheet with nonstick cooking spray. Scrub a potato, then slice it into $1/4$-inch-thick slices. (The skin can be left on or removed.) Distribute the potato slices in a single layer over the cookie sheet. Bake until crisp, about 15 minutes. (Watch closely so that they don't burn.) Add salt and pepper to taste.

my goal(s) for this week:

_____
_____
_____

Things that might trip me up:

_____
_____
_____

How I plan to deal with them:

_____
_____
_____

MY PLAN FOR EXERCISE/PHYSICAL ACTIVITY

Type of activity/length of time   **What I actually did**

Sunday:_____   _____

Monday:_____   _____

Tuesday:_____   _____

Wednesday:_____   _____

Thursday:_____   _____

Friday:_____   _____

Saturday:_____   _____

Daily Diary

Date: _____

Hunger: 1 = starving
2 = kind of hungry
3 = not hungry

Foods, beverages & snacks I had today:

	Food or beverage and amount	Hunger	Calories/Other	Feelings/Mood
MORNING				
AFTERNOON				
EVENING				
DAILY TOTAL				

Exercise/Physical activities:

Plan for tomorrow:

Today's successes/Random thoughts:

Daily Diary

Date: _____

Foods, beverages & snacks I had today:

	Food or beverage and amount	Hunger	Calories/Other	Feelings/Mood
MORNING				
AFTERNOON				
EVENING				
DAILY TOTAL				

Exercise/Physical activities:	Plan for tomorrow:

Today's successes/Random thoughts:

Daily Diary

Date: _____

Foods, beverages & snacks I had today:

	Food or beverage and amount	Hunger	Calories/Other	Feelings/Mood
MORNING				
AFTERNOON				
EVENING				
DAILY TOTAL				

Exercise/Physical activities:

Plan for tomorrow:

Today's successes/Random thoughts:

Daily Diary

Date:_____

Foods, beverages & snacks I had today:

	Food or beverage and amount	Hunger	Calories/ Other	Feelings/Mood
MORNING				
AFTERNOON				
EVENING				
DAILY TOTAL				

Exercise/Physical activities:	Plan for tomorrow:

Today's successes/Random thoughts:

Daily Diary

Date:_____

Foods, beverages & snacks I had today:

	Food or beverage and amount	Hunger	Calories/ Other	Feelings/Mood
MORNING				
AFTERNOON				
EVENING				
DAILY TOTAL				

Exercise/Physical activities:

Plan for tomorrow:

Today's successes/Random thoughts:

Daily Diary

Date: _____

Hunger: 1 = starving
2 = kind of hungry
3 = not hungry

Foods, beverages & snacks I had today:

	Food or beverage and amount	Hunger	Calories/Other	Feelings/Mood
MORNING				
AFTERNOON				
EVENING				
DAILY TOTAL				

Exercise/Physical activities:

Plan for tomorrow:

Today's successes/Random thoughts:

Daily Diary

Date: _____

Hunger: 1 = starving
2 = kind of hungry
3 = not hungry

Foods, beverages & snacks I had today:

	Food or beverage and amount	Hunger	Calories/Other	Feelings/Mood
MORNING				
AFTERNOON				
EVENING				
DAILY TOTAL				

Exercise/Physical activities:

Plan for tomorrow:

Today's successes/Random thoughts:

Review of My Week

Things that really helped this week:

_____
_____
_____

Was/Were my goal(s) met?

_____
_____
_____

I'd like to work on this:

_____
_____
_____

Reminders of why I want to get to a healthier weight:

_____
_____
_____

Reminders of how my life is better already:

_____
_____
_____

MY WEIGHT:_____

MY SPACE

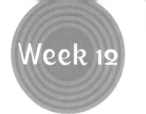

Week 12

Be realistic about your weight goal.

"I'm not going to be a skinny person. I thought I was for a minute, but I'm not. It's genetics — everyone in my family has big hips. This is the way I am. If someone doesn't like it, oh well! As long as I keep maintaining, I'm okay."

— Robin S.

About Robin: The most Robin ever weighed was 170 pounds, when she was 9 years old and 5'3". At 13, she's grown to 5'6" and weighs 150.

Habits before: "I used to come home, do homework, and watch TV." She also ate too much "Southern food," like fried pork chops.

Turning point: "I was tired of having people tease me, and I wasn't happy with myself."

How she did it: "I went to Weight Watchers with my godmother and started to pay attention to what I was eating. Being active was important too." Now she eats more vegetables, watches portion sizes, drinks less soda and more water, and goes easy on fast foods and snack foods. She says, "I stay focused on what my goals are and try not to let others distract me."

How she stays fit: "I'm on the school basketball team and we practice 3 days a week for 2 to 3 hours. I'm also a cheerleader and have practice 2 days a week."

How can YOU be realistic about your weight goal?

Recognize how far you've come. Emily B. says, "Think about what you were like before you lost the weight. Accept that you've already done something really hard and that you're in the weight range that's healthy and natural. Be happy that you've come so far and enjoy how much better you feel."

Focus on things you like about yourself, aside from your appearance. Kristy C. says, "Don't fret over nitpicky things like cellulite and a few extra inches in the thighs. Try to focus on what you love about yourself instead. Make a list of these things and read it when you feel lonely or depressed."

wlcj

Make a list of the things you like about yourself.

_____

_____

_____

_____

_____

_____

_____

_____

_____

my goal(s) for this week:

_____

_____

_____

Things that might trip me up:

_____

_____

_____

How I plan to deal with them:

_____

_____

_____

MY PLAN FOR EXERCISE/PHYSICAL ACTIVITY

Type of activity/length of time

What I actually did

Sunday:_____   _____

Monday:_____   _____

Tuesday:_____   _____

Wednesday:_____   _____

Thursday:_____   _____

Friday:_____   _____

Saturday:_____   _____

Daily Diary

Date: _____

Hunger: 1 = starving
2 = kind of hungry
3 = not hungry

Foods, beverages & snacks I had today:

	Food or beverage and amount	Hunger	Calories/Other	Feelings/Mood
MORNING				
AFTERNOON				
EVENING				
DAILY TOTAL				

Exercise/Physical activities:	Plan for tomorrow:

Today's successes/Random thoughts:

Daily Diary

Date:_____

Hunger: 1 = starving
2 = kind of hungry
3 = not hungry

Foods, beverages & snacks I had today:

	Food or beverage and amount	Hunger	Calories/Other	Feelings/Mood
MORNING				
AFTERNOON				
EVENING				
DAILY TOTAL				

Exercise/Physical activities:	Plan for tomorrow:

Today's successes/Random thoughts:

Daily Diary

Date: _____

Foods, beverages & snacks I had today:

Food or beverage and amount	Hunger	Calories/Other	Feelings/Mood
MORNING			
AFTERNOON			
EVENING			
DAILY TOTAL			

Exercise/Physical activities:

Plan for tomorrow:

Today's successes/Random thoughts:

Daily Diary

Date:_____

Foods, beverages & snacks I had today:

	Food or beverage and amount	Hunger	Calories/ Other	Feelings/Mood
MORNING				
AFTERNOON				
EVENING				
	DAILY TOTAL			

Exercise/Physical activities:	Plan for tomorrow:

Today's successes/Random thoughts:

Daily Diary

Date: _____

Hunger: 1 = starving
2 = kind of hungry
3 = not hungry

Foods, beverages & snacks I had today:

Food or beverage and amount	Hunger	Calories/Other	Feelings/Mood
DAILY TOTAL			

MORNING

AFTERNOON

EVENING

Exercise/Physical activities:

Plan for tomorrow:

Today's successes/Random thoughts:

Daily Diary

Date:_____

Foods, beverages & snacks I had today:

	Food or beverage and amount	Hunger	Calories/Other	Feelings/Mood
MORNING				
AFTERNOON				
EVENING				
	DAILY TOTAL			

Exercise/Physical activities:	Plan for tomorrow:

Today's successes/Random thoughts:

Daily Diary

Date: _____

Foods, beverages & snacks I had today:

	Food or beverage and amount	Hunger	Calories/Other	Feelings/Mood
MORNING				
AFTERNOON				
EVENING				
DAILY TOTAL				

Exercise/Physical activities:

Plan for tomorrow:

Today's successes/Random thoughts:

Review of My Week

Things that really helped this week:

_____
_____
_____

Was/Were my goal(s) met?

_____
_____
_____

I'd like to work on this:

_____
_____
_____

Reminders of why I want to get to a healthier weight:

_____
_____
_____

Reminders of how my life is better already:

_____
_____
_____

MY WEIGHT:_____

MY SPACE

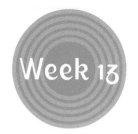

Week 13 Get your family to help you get rid of temptations.

> "If tempting foods are around, you feel like your family's not supporting your ambitions. When you're home, you want to relax and not have to worry about being tempted."
>
> — Kristen F.

About Kristen: When Kristen started slimming down, she was almost 12, weighed 150, and was 5' tall. Now 15, she's 5'5" and weighs 148 pounds.

Habits before: Too much snacking. "There were always candy, cookies, chips, and sugar drinks in the house."

Turning point: Kristen was tired of the way other teens treated her. "I was like a beaten dog. I wanted to show them all that I was better than what they said."

How she did it: She went to Camp Shane, a weight loss camp. When she got home, she worked with her mom to stock the kitchen with healthy foods rather than sweets and high-calorie snack foods. "I eat no fried foods, drink no soda pop, have smaller portions, and eat frequent small snacks of fruits, juices, and skim milk." She treats herself to ice cream once in a while but no longer feels she has to order dessert every time she goes out to eat.

How she stays fit: "I dance 3 days a week for 30 minutes, stretch 6 days a week for 10 minutes, and walk 3 days a week for 40 minutes."

How can you get your family to help you get rid of temptations?

"Parents need to understand that having tons of junk food around is practically sabotage," says Mary N. The teens and their parents also said that it's important for the entire family to try to eat healthier foods — not just the family members who are overweight.

When Zach G.'s mother buys sweets, he either asks her to stop buying them or tells her to hide them.

Make a list of ways your family can help you — for instance, by buying more fruits and vegetables and having them washed and cut up, buying less high-calorie snack food, having dessert just once a week, doing less baking, buying more low-fat foods, or switching to diet soda or flavored water. Consider sharing the list with your family.

_____

_____

_____

_____

RICHIE C.'S SPINACH WITH GARLIC
Heat 1 tablespoon olive oil in a large nonstick pan over medium heat. Add a few thinly sliced garlic cloves and cook for a minute or two. Add $1/2$ c. chicken broth and a bag of fresh, washed spinach. Cover and cook until spinach is wilted. If desired, top with fresh-squeezed lemon juice, plus salt and pepper to taste.

my goal(s) for this week:

_____

_____

_____

Things that might trip me up:

_____

_____

_____

How I plan to deal with them:

_____

_____

_____

MY PLAN FOR EXERCISE/PHYSICAL ACTIVITY

Type of activity/length of time

What I actually did

Sunday:_____   _____

Monday:_____   _____

Tuesday:_____   _____

Wednesday:_____   _____

Thursday:_____   _____

Friday:_____   _____

Saturday:_____   _____

Daily Diary

Date: _____

Hunger: 1 = starving
2 = kind of hungry
3 = not hungry

Foods, beverages & snacks I had today:

	Food or beverage and amount	Hunger	Calories/Other	Feelings/Mood
MORNING				
AFTERNOON				
EVENING				
DAILY TOTAL				

Exercise/Physical activities:

Plan for tomorrow:

Today's successes/Random thoughts:

Daily Diary

Date:_____

Hunger: 1 = starving
2 = kind of hungry
3 = not hungry

Foods, beverages & snacks I had today:

	Food or beverage and amount	Hunger	Calories/Other	Feelings/Mood
MORNING				
AFTERNOON				
EVENING				
DAILY TOTAL				

Exercise/Physical activities:	Plan for tomorrow:

Today's successes/Random thoughts:

Daily Diary

Date: _____

Hunger: 1 = starving
2 = kind of hungry
3 = not hungry

Foods, beverages & snacks I had today:

	Food or beverage and amount	Hunger	Calories/Other	Feelings/Mood
MORNING				
AFTERNOON				
EVENING				
DAILY TOTAL				

Exercise/Physical activities:

Plan for tomorrow:

Today's successes/Random thoughts:

Daily Diary

Date:_____

Foods, beverages & snacks I had today:

	Food or beverage and amount	Hunger	Calories/Other	Feelings/Mood
MORNING				
AFTERNOON				
EVENING				
DAILY TOTAL				

Exercise/Physical activities:	Plan for tomorrow:

Today's successes/Random thoughts:

Daily Diary

Date: _____

Foods, beverages & snacks I had today:

Food or beverage and amount	Hunger	Calories/Other	Feelings/Mood
MORNING			
AFTERNOON			
EVENING			
DAILY TOTAL			

Exercise/Physical activities:

Plan for tomorrow:

Today's successes/Random thoughts:

Daily Diary

Date: _____

Hunger: 1 = starving
2 = kind of hungry
3 = not hungry

Foods, beverages & snacks I had today:

	Food or beverage and amount	Hunger	Calories/Other	Feelings/Mood
MORNING				
AFTERNOON				
EVENING				
DAILY TOTAL				

Exercise/Physical activities:	Plan for tomorrow:

Today's successes/Random thoughts:

Daily Diary

Date: _____

Hunger: 1 = starving
2 = kind of hungry
3 = not hungry

Foods, beverages & snacks I had today:

	Food or beverage and amount	Hunger	Calories/Other	Feelings/Mood
MORNING				
AFTERNOON				
EVENING				
DAILY TOTAL				

Exercise/Physical activities:

Plan for tomorrow:

Today's successes/Random thoughts:

Review of My Week

Things that really helped this week:

_____
_____
_____

Was/Were my goal(s) met?

_____
_____
_____

I'd like to work on this:

_____
_____
_____

Reminders of why I want to get to a healthier weight:

_____
_____
_____

Reminders of how my life is better already:

_____
_____
_____

MY WEIGHT:_____

MY SPACE

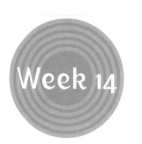

Find ways to stick with exercise.

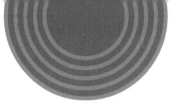

"By scheduling exercise, I increase the chances that I will work out. And since I get bored with doing the same thing every day, I keep things fun by doing whatever exercise I feel like. If you have fun when you work out, you start looking forward to it instead of viewing it as a chore."

— Paula D.

About Paula: "I went through what I call my 'fat years' from 8th through 12th grades." Paula's highest weight was 170, when she was 5'5" tall. At 19, as a college student, she slimmed down to 140, a weight she's maintained for more than 3½ years. (She's 5'7" now.)

Habits before: Paula's biggest problem was not getting enough exercise.

Turning point: "When regular sizes no longer fit, I didn't want to have to wear plus sizes."

How she did it: The most important change was exercising. "At first, I swam with my roommate, who was also overweight. Then I started going to workout classes at my college gym." After losing the weight, she says she still eats the same number of meals and snacks as she did when she was heavier — but now her portion sizes are smaller. When she visits her parents, Paula says, "I refuse to eat out every night with them."

How she stays fit: "I do step aerobics for 30 minutes 3 times a week. Sometimes, instead of a step class, I swim for 45 minutes. I also do some hip-hop dancing, kickboxing, and yoga. Exercise keeps the stress down, so I do less stress eating."

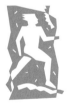

How can you stick with exercise?

Rose Q.: "When I'm in a rut with my workouts, I'll either try a new group class or do things outside, like go for walks and runs or go to a playground."

Christine F.: "Exercise can suck at first — you're tired, sweaty, and in some pain. Then a few weeks pass, and you see results. As soon as there were visible rewards, I was hooked."

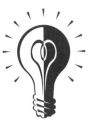

Think about ways you can stick with exercise — for instance, by scheduling it, finding ways to make it fun, varying what you do on different days, or trying something new.

_____
_____

What payback do you get from exercising?

_____
_____
_____
_____
_____

try this:

MATTHEW L.'S FAVORITE BREAKFAST
Oatmeal, cooked in the microwave and topped with a little brown sugar or real maple syrup.

my goal(s) for this week:

_____
_____
_____

Things that might trip me up:

_____
_____
_____

How I plan to deal with them:

_____
_____
_____

MY PLAN FOR EXERCISE/PHYSICAL ACTIVITY

Type of activity/length of time   What I actually did

Sunday:_____   _____

Monday:_____   _____

Tuesday:_____   _____

Wednesday:_____   _____

Thursday:_____   _____

Friday:_____   _____

Saturday:_____   _____

Daily Diary

Date: _____

Hunger: 1 = starving
2 = kind of hungry
3 = not hungry

Foods, beverages & snacks I had today:

	Food or beverage and amount	Hunger	Calories/Other	Feelings/Mood
MORNING				
AFTERNOON				
EVENING				
DAILY TOTAL				

Exercise/Physical activities:

Plan for tomorrow:

Today's successes/Random thoughts:

Daily Diary

Date: _____

Hunger: 1 = starving
2 = kind of hungry
3 = not hungry

Foods, beverages & snacks I had today:

	Food or beverage and amount	Hunger	Calories/ Other	Feelings/Mood
MORNING				
AFTERNOON				
EVENING				
DAILY TOTAL				

Exercise/Physical activities:	Plan for tomorrow:

Today's successes/Random thoughts:

Daily Diary

Date: _____

Foods, beverages & snacks I had today:

	Food or beverage and amount	Hunger	Calories/Other	Feelings/Mood
MORNING				
AFTERNOON				
EVENING				
DAILY TOTAL				

Exercise/Physical activities:	Plan for tomorrow:

Today's successes/Random thoughts:

Daily Diary

Date: _____

Foods, beverages & snacks I had today:

	Food or beverage and amount	Hunger	Calories/Other	Feelings/Mood
MORNING				
AFTERNOON				
EVENING				
	DAILY TOTAL			

Exercise/Physical activities:	Plan for tomorrow:

Today's successes/Random thoughts:

Daily Diary

Date: _____

Foods, beverages & snacks I had today:

	Food or beverage and amount	Hunger	Calories/ Other	Feelings/Mood
MORNING				
AFTERNOON				
EVENING				
DAILY TOTAL				

Exercise/Physical activities:	Plan for tomorrow:

Today's successes/Random thoughts:

Daily Diary

Date: _____

Foods, beverages & snacks I had today:

	Food or beverage and amount	Hunger	Calories/ Other	Feelings/Mood
MORNING				
AFTERNOON				
EVENING				
DAILY TOTAL				

Exercise/Physical activities:	Plan for tomorrow:

Today's successes/Random thoughts:

Daily Diary

Date:_____

Hunger: 1 = starving
2 = kind of hungry
3 = not hungry

Foods, beverages & snacks I had today:

Food or beverage and amount	Hunger	Calories/Other	Feelings/Mood
MORNING			
AFTERNOON			
EVENING			
DAILY TOTAL			

Exercise/Physical activities:	Plan for tomorrow:

Today's successes/Random thoughts:

Review of My Week

Things that really helped this week:

_____

_____

_____

Was/Were my goal(s) met?

_____

_____

_____

I'd like to work on this:

_____

_____

_____

Reminders of why I want to get to a healthier weight:

_____

_____

_____

Reminders of how my life is better already:

_____

_____

_____

MY WEIGHT:_____

MY SPACE

Tune in to your body's hunger signals.

"I eat only when my stomach feels kind of empty and I feel hunger pangs. Instead of eating till I'm full, I eat just until I satisfy the empty feeling, not until I'm uncomfortable and can't eat anymore."

— Ethan Q.

About Ethan: At 240 pounds, Ethan hit his highest weight when he was 5'10". He decided to lose weight at 15. He's 16 now, stands 6'2", and weighs 190 pounds.

Habits before: "I'd keep eating and eating. It was like a constant hunger when I was bored, even though I knew I wasn't really hungry."

Turning point: "I didn't have many friends, and I was tired of being picked on. I hated not being able to do physical activities with my brothers."

How he did it: Ethan went to a kids' summer weight program at Camp La Jolla. "The friends who lost weight with me kept me motivated." One of his most important strategies when he got home was "keeping busy."

How he stays fit: "I do cardio on an elliptical machine and running for at least an hour, 5 days a week." He also lifts weights every day.

FIVE STRATEGIES FROM TEENS
How can you tune in to your body's hunger signals?

1. Is your stomach growling? Do you have an empty feeling? Has it been a few hours since you last ate?
2. Really pay attention to what you're eating.
3. After eating a reasonable amount of food, ask yourself, "If I keep on eating, will I feel stuffed?"
4. Have a glass of water or no-cal beverage — then see whether you're still hungry.

5. Ethan Q. says, "Slowing down when I eat gives my stomach time to catch up."

What's your strategy for tuning in to your hunger?

_____
_____
_____
_____
_____

try this:

LEE J.'S TEX-MEX POTATO
Prick a baking potato in a few places with a fork and microwave until it is soft in the middle. Cut it open and top with some salsa, a tablespoon or two of light or fat-free sour cream, and some black beans.

my goal(s) for this week:

_____
_____
_____

Things that might trip me up:

_____
_____
_____

How I plan to deal with them:

_____
_____
_____

MY PLAN FOR EXERCISE/PHYSICAL ACTIVITY

Type of activity/length of time

What I actually did

Sunday:_____   _____

Monday:_____   _____

Tuesday:_____   _____

Wednesday:_____   _____

Thursday:_____   _____

Friday:_____   _____

Saturday:_____   _____

Daily Diary

Date: _____

Hunger: 1 = starving
2 = kind of hungry
3 = not hungry

Foods, beverages & snacks I had today:

	Food or beverage and amount	Hunger	Calories/Other	Feelings/Mood
MORNING				
AFTERNOON				
EVENING				
DAILY TOTAL				

Exercise/Physical activities:

Plan for tomorrow:

Today's successes/Random thoughts:

Daily Diary

Date: _____

Foods, beverages & snacks I had today:

	Food or beverage and amount	Hunger	Calories/Other	Feelings/Mood
MORNING				
AFTERNOON				
EVENING				
DAILY TOTAL				

Exercise/Physical activities:	Plan for tomorrow:

Today's successes/Random thoughts:

Daily Diary

Date: _____

Foods, beverages & snacks I had today:

Food or beverage and amount	Hunger	Calories/Other	Feelings/Mood
MORNING			
AFTERNOON			
EVENING			
DAILY TOTAL			

Exercise/Physical activities:	Plan for tomorrow:

Today's successes/Random thoughts:

Daily Diary

Date: _____

Foods, beverages & snacks I had today:

Food or beverage and amount	Hunger	Calories/Other	Feelings/Mood
MORNING			
AFTERNOON			
EVENING			
DAILY TOTAL			

Exercise/Physical activities:	Plan for tomorrow:

Today's successes/Random thoughts:

Daily Diary

Date:_____

Hunger: 1 = starving
2 = kind of hungry
3 = not hungry

Foods, beverages & snacks I had today:

	Food or beverage and amount	Hunger	Calories/Other	Feelings/Mood
MORNING				
AFTERNOON				
EVENING				
DAILY TOTAL				

Exercise/Physical activities:	Plan for tomorrow:

Today's successes/Random thoughts:

Daily Diary

Date: _____

Foods, beverages & snacks I had today:

	Food or beverage and amount	Hunger	Calories/Other	Feelings/Mood
MORNING				
AFTERNOON				
EVENING				
	DAILY TOTAL			

Exercise/Physical activities:	Plan for tomorrow:

Today's successes/Random thoughts:

Daily Diary

Date:_____

Hunger: 1 = starving
2 = kind of hungry
3 = not hungry

Foods, beverages & snacks I had today:

Food or beverage and amount	Hunger	Calories/ Other	Feelings/Mood

MORNING

AFTERNOON

EVENING

| DAILY TOTAL | | | |

Exercise/Physical activities:

Plan for tomorrow:

Today's successes/Random thoughts:

Review of My Week

Things that really helped this week:

_____
_____
_____

Was/Were my goal(s) met?

_____
_____
_____

I'd like to work on this:

_____
_____
_____

Reminders of why I want to get to a healthier weight:

_____
_____
_____

Reminders of how my life is better already:

_____
_____
_____

MY WEIGHT:_____

MY SPACE

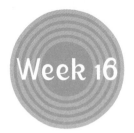

Week 16

Cut your "seat time."

About Kristy: Kristy's highest weight was 145, which she hit when she was 12 and just 5 feet tall. She started losing sometime between 7th and 8th grades. She's now 21, is 5'5", and weighs 140.

Habits before: "Despite going to sports practices and dance classes, I spent a lot of my free time in front of the TV."

Turning point: Kristy says her main incentive was wanting to improve her appearance and health.

How she did it: "I happened upon an exercise regime that I really loved — dancing and doing video step classes at home — which led me to learn more about healthy eating." Today, she says, "I make an active decision to eat well, enjoying fruits and vegetables and trying to balance out my carbohydrates with protein and fat. I allow myself to indulge but try to keep it to a minimum, like a piece of chocolate instead of a whole bar or bag."

How she stays fit: "I exercise almost every day. Each week, I do 2 hours of kickboxing, 3 hours of step classes, and 2 hours of weightlifting."

> "Filling my schedule helped me get my butt off the couch. That way, when I wasn't in school, I was at some afterschool activity. I didn't have as much time for TV, which meant I wasn't snacking as much either."
>
> — Kristy C.

How can you cut your "seat time"?

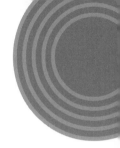

Get involved in extracurricular activities. Kristy "padded" her schedule so that she had less time to watch TV.

Set a time limit for TV and computer and video game time and stick to it — no more than 2 hours a day.

Be selective. "Now I don't just sit in front of the TV. I generally watch only specific shows." — Alyssa M.

Watch TV while working out. "It keeps my mind off how much time I have left in my workout." — Sandra D.

Be more active.

Walk to the store, work, or classes instead of driving or taking the bus.

Take the stairs instead of escalators or elevators.

Park your car in the farthest spot away from the mall, school, or wherever you're going.

wlcj

162

Do physical activity first. "I don't turn on the TV until I've gone for a walk, gone to the gym, or done some form of exercise — even if it's only 10 minutes." — Margaret G.

try this:

SEAN C.'S CHILI
Heat a serving of canned vegetarian chili in a small pan or a microwavable bowl. Top with some fat-free sour cream and a sprinkling of shredded low-fat cheddar cheese.

 For a few days this week, keep a record of how much time you spend in front of the TV or the computer.

Sunday _____ hours   Monday _____ hours   Tuesday _____ hours
Wednesday _____ hours   Thursday _____ hours   Friday _____ hours
Saturday _____ hours

my goal(s) for this week:

_____
_____
_____

Things that might trip me up: How I plan to deal with them:

_____   _____
_____   _____
_____   _____

MY PLAN FOR EXERCISE/PHYSICAL ACTIVITY

Type of activity/length of time   What I actually did

Sunday:_____   _____

Monday:_____   _____

Tuesday:_____   _____

Wednesday:_____   _____

Thursday:_____   _____

Friday:_____   _____

Saturday:_____   _____

Daily Diary

Date:_____

Hunger: 1 = starving
2 = kind of hungry
3 = not hungry

Foods, beverages & snacks I had today:

	Food or beverage and amount	Hunger	Calories/Other	Feelings/Mood
MORNING				
AFTERNOON				
EVENING				
DAILY TOTAL				

Exercise/Physical activities:

Plan for tomorrow:

Today's successes/Random thoughts:

Daily Diary

Date:_____

Hunger: 1 = starving
2 = kind of hungry
3 = not hungry

Foods, beverages & snacks I had today:

	Food or beverage and amount	Hunger	Calories/Other	Feelings/Mood
MORNING				
AFTERNOON				
EVENING				
DAILY TOTAL				

Exercise/Physical activities:	Plan for tomorrow:

Today's successes/Random thoughts:

week 16 — day 2   165

Daily Diary

Date:_____

Foods, beverages & snacks I had today:

	Food or beverage and amount	Hunger	Calories/ Other	Feelings/Mood
MORNING				
AFTERNOON				
EVENING				
DAILY TOTAL				

Exercise/Physical activities:	Plan for tomorrow:

Today's successes/Random thoughts:

Daily Diary

Date:_____

Foods, beverages & snacks I had today:

	Food or beverage and amount	Hunger	Calories/Other	Feelings/Mood
MORNING				
AFTERNOON				
EVENING				
DAILY TOTAL				

Exercise/Physical activities:	Plan for tomorrow:

Today's successes/Random thoughts:

Daily Diary

Date:_____

Foods, beverages & snacks I had today:

	Food or beverage and amount	Hunger	Calories/Other	Feelings/Mood
MORNING				
AFTERNOON				
EVENING				
DAILY TOTAL				

Exercise/Physical activities:

Plan for tomorrow:

Today's successes/Random thoughts:

Daily Diary

Date: _____

Hunger: 1 = starving
2 = kind of hungry
3 = not hungry

Foods, beverages & snacks I had today:

	Food or beverage and amount	Hunger	Calories/Other	Feelings/Mood
MORNING				
AFTERNOON				
EVENING				
DAILY TOTAL				

Exercise/Physical activities:

Plan for tomorrow:

Today's successes/Random thoughts:

Daily Diary

Date: _____

Foods, beverages & snacks I had today:

	Food or beverage and amount	Hunger	Calories/Other	Feelings/Mood
MORNING				
AFTERNOON				
EVENING				
DAILY TOTAL				

Exercise/Physical activities:	Plan for tomorrow:

Today's successes/Random thoughts:

Review of My Week

□ Things that really helped this week:
_____
_____
_____

□ Was/Were my goal(s) met?
_____
_____
_____

□ I'd like to work on this:
_____
_____
_____

□ Reminders of why I want to get to a healthier weight:
_____
_____
_____

□ Reminders of how my life is better already:
_____
_____
_____

MY WEIGHT:_____

MY SPACE

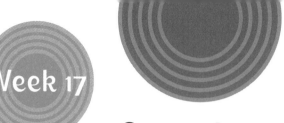

Week 17

Snack smarter.

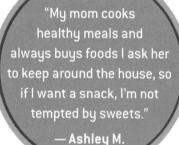

"My mom cooks healthy meals and always buys foods I ask her to keep around the house, so if I want a snack, I'm not tempted by sweets."

— **Ashley M.**

About Ashley: Her heaviest weight was 250 pounds, when she was 5'4". At 16, she started slimming down. She's now 17, weighs 148, and is 5'5".

Habits before: "I used to snack and not eat regular meals."

Turning point: "My twin sister had seen a nutritionist and encouraged me to meet with her too. I didn't want to go because I had tried other programs that didn't work. But I saw my sister's success and liked the nutritionist, so I gave it a try."

How she did it: Both Ashley and her sister saw the dietitian/nutritionist for one-on-one counseling every week. Because the approach was different for each one, they had their own separate appointments. Ashley hated to exercise, so her initial focus was on eating fewer sugary foods. She kept food records for about four months; after that, she'd keep track of what she ate only when she was having trouble losing weight. Eventually, she started walking and also rode an exercise bike. She eats regular meals (a morning snack, lunch, and dinner) and makes healthier restaurant and snack choices. She says having protein throughout the day helps her feel full and snack less often.

How she stays fit: She walks 30 to 45 minutes with her dog each day and tries to ride the exercise bike for 45 minutes 4 days a week.

try these:

JAYDEN L.'S FAVORITE LOWER-CALORIE TREATS
97 percent fat-free kettle corn; TCBY soft serve frozen yogurt; The Skinny Cow ice cream sandwiches; fat-free, sugar-free pudding with fat-free Cool Whip.

TYLER D.'S HAM AND CREAM CHEESE ROLL-UPS
Spread a tortilla with some fat-free cream cheese and top with 1 or 2 thin slices of lean ham. Roll it up.

How can you snack smarter?

Rose Q.: "Rice cakes and those Light & Fit Smoothies are great snacks."

Marie P.: "If I want something sweet, I'll have peanut butter on celery or an apple, or I have baby carrots and low-fat salad dressing."

Sid J.: "I switched to a lower-fat microwave popcorn. At the movie theater, I ask for an extra empty box and give half away."

Katie S.: "I eat one or two snacks a day, ranging from hummus on pita bread to yogurt or fruit to a controlled portion of kettle chips."

Make a list of healthy, quick snacks that will work for you.

_____

_____

_____

my goal(s) for this week:

_____

_____

_____

Things that might trip me up: How I plan to deal with them:

_____   _____

_____   _____

_____   _____

MY PLAN FOR EXERCISE/PHYSICAL ACTIVITY

Type of activity/length of time   What I actually did

Sunday:_____   _____

Monday:_____   _____

Tuesday:_____   _____

Wednesday:_____   _____

Thursday:_____   _____

Friday:_____   _____

Saturday:_____   _____

Daily Diary

Date: _____

Hunger: 1 = starving
2 = kind of hungry
3 = not hungry

Foods, beverages & snacks I had today:

	Food or beverage and amount	Hunger	Calories/Other	Feelings/Mood
MORNING				
AFTERNOON				
EVENING				
	DAILY TOTAL			

Exercise/Physical activities:

Plan for tomorrow:

Today's successes/Random thoughts:

Daily Diary

Date: _____

Hunger: 1 = starving
2 = kind of hungry
3 = not hungry

Foods, beverages & snacks I had today:

	Food or beverage and amount	Hunger	Calories/Other	Feelings/Mood
MORNING				
AFTERNOON				
EVENING				
	DAILY TOTAL			

Exercise/Physical activities:	Plan for tomorrow:

Today's successes/Random thoughts:

week 17 — day 2   175

Daily Diary

Date: _____

Hunger: 1 = starving
2 = kind of hungry
3 = not hungry

Foods, beverages & snacks I had today:

	Food or beverage and amount	Hunger	Calories/Other	Feelings/Mood
MORNING				
AFTERNOON				
EVENING				
DAILY TOTAL				

Exercise/Physical activities:

Plan for tomorrow:

Today's successes/Random thoughts:

Daily Diary

Date:_____

Hunger: 1 = starving
2 = kind of hungry
3 = not hungry

Foods, beverages & snacks I had today:

	Food or beverage and amount	Hunger	Calories/Other	Feelings/Mood
MORNING				
AFTERNOON				
EVENING				
DAILY TOTAL				

Exercise/Physical activities:	Plan for tomorrow:

Today's successes/Random thoughts:

Daily Diary

Date: _____

Hunger: 1 = starving
2 = kind of hungry
3 = not hungry

Foods, beverages & snacks I had today:

	Food or beverage and amount	Hunger	Calories/ Other	Feelings/Mood
MORNING				
AFTERNOON				
EVENING				
DAILY TOTAL				

Exercise/Physical activities:

Plan for tomorrow:

Today's successes/Random thoughts:

Daily Diary

Date: _____

Hunger: 1 = starving
         2 = kind of hungry
         3 = not hungry

Foods, beverages & snacks I had today:

	Food or beverage and amount	Hunger	Calories/Other	Feelings/Mood
MORNING				
AFTERNOON				
EVENING				
DAILY TOTAL				

Exercise/Physical activities:	Plan for tomorrow:

Today's successes/Random thoughts:

Daily Diary

Date: _____

Hunger: 1 = starving
2 = kind of hungry
3 = not hungry

Foods, beverages & snacks I had today:

	Food or beverage and amount	Hunger	Calories/Other	Feelings/Mood
MORNING				
AFTERNOON				
EVENING				
DAILY TOTAL				

Exercise/Physical activities:

Plan for tomorrow:

Today's successes/Random thoughts:

Review of My Week

▣ Things that really helped this week:

_____

_____

_____

▣ Was/Were my goal(s) met?

_____

_____

_____

▣ I'd like to work on this:

_____

_____

_____

▣ Reminders of why I want to get to a healthier weight:

_____

_____

_____

▣ Reminders of how my life is better already:

_____

_____

_____

MY WEIGHT:_____

MY SPACE

Get a grip on emotional overeating.

"Eating for emotional reasons makes you feel better for only a short time. Exercise helps me more than eating does."

— Felicia S.

About Felicia: By the time she was 13, she'd reached 180 pounds and was 5'6". About a year and a half ago, she started losing weight. She's now 15½, weighs 139, and has grown an inch.

Habits before: Felicia's weight gain started when her parents were going through a divorce. Not long after that, her mother died. "Food was one of the few things I enjoyed at the time, and I'm sure I ate to push my thoughts away."

Turning point: "I wanted to fit into clothes and look good in them."

How she did it: She went to a kids' summer weight program at Camp La Jolla and says, "When I returned from camp, I ate a more balanced diet. Portion control was a huge factor — I continued to eat most foods, just less of them. I also avoided foods high in fat, would eat only when truly hungry, and joined a gym. Now I make sure what I'm eating is really worth it. And before I go to a restaurant, I set my mind on what I'm going to eat."

How she stays fit: "I rollerblade for 45 to 60 minutes 4 or 5 days a week. Occasionally, I go on an elliptical trainer for 45 minutes."

How can YOU start to get a grip on emotional overeating?

Try Kristy C.'s strategy: "I evaluate my eating motivations — hunger versus boredom, for example." She suggests asking yourself: "Why do I feel the need to eat right now? Am I lonely? Do I feel like some aspect of my life is out of control? How will eating solve this problem?"

Several teens said that keeping a journal is a good way to channel emotions, and a number of them find that it helps to talk with a friend or other supportive person.

Think about your reasons for emotional overeating and list some strategies that might help you cope.

_____
_____
_____
_____
_____
_____
_____
_____

my goal(s) for this week:

_____
_____
_____

Things that might trip me up:

_____
_____
_____

How I plan to deal with them:

_____
_____
_____

MY PLAN FOR EXERCISE/PHYSICAL ACTIVITY

Type of activity/length of time

What I actually did

Sunday:_____   _____

Monday:_____   _____

Tuesday:_____   _____

Wednesday:_____   _____

Thursday:_____   _____

Friday:_____   _____

Saturday:_____   _____

Daily Diary

Date:_____

Hunger: 1 = starving
2 = kind of hungry
3 = not hungry

Foods, beverages & snacks I had today:

	Food or beverage and amount	Hunger	Calories/Other	Feelings/Mood
MORNING				
AFTERNOON				
EVENING				
DAILY TOTAL				

Exercise/Physical activities:	Plan for tomorrow:

Today's successes/Random thoughts:

Daily Diary

Date:_____

Foods, beverages & snacks I had today:

	Food or beverage and amount	Hunger	Calories/Other	Feelings/Mood
MORNING				
AFTERNOON				
EVENING				
	DAILY TOTAL			

Exercise/Physical activities:	Plan for tomorrow:

Today's successes/Random thoughts:

Daily Diary

Date: _____

Foods, beverages & snacks I had today:

	Food or beverage and amount	Hunger	Calories/Other	Feelings/Mood
MORNING				
AFTERNOON				
EVENING				
DAILY TOTAL				

Exercise/Physical activities:

Plan for tomorrow:

Today's successes/Random thoughts:

Daily Diary

Date: _____

Foods, beverages & snacks I had today:

	Food or beverage and amount	Hunger	Calories/ Other	Feelings/Mood
MORNING				
AFTERNOON				
EVENING				
DAILY TOTAL				

Exercise/Physical activities:

Plan for tomorrow:

Today's successes/Random thoughts:

Daily Diary

Date:_____

Foods, beverages & snacks I had today:

	Food or beverage and amount	Hunger	Calories/ Other	Feelings/Mood
MORNING				
AFTERNOON				
EVENING				
DAILY TOTAL				

Exercise/Physical activities:	Plan for tomorrow:

Today's successes/Random thoughts:

Daily Diary

Date: _____

Hunger: 1 = starving
2 = kind of hungry
3 = not hungry

Foods, beverages & snacks I had today:

	Food or beverage and amount	Hunger	Calories/Other	Feelings/Mood
MORNING				
AFTERNOON				
EVENING				
DAILY TOTAL				

Exercise/Physical activities:

Plan for tomorrow:

Today's successes/Random thoughts:

Daily Diary

Date: _____

Hunger: 1 = starving
2 = kind of hungry
3 = not hungry

Foods, beverages & snacks I had today:

	Food or beverage and amount	Hunger	Calories/Other	Feelings/Mood
MORNING				
AFTERNOON				
EVENING				
	DAILY TOTAL			

Exercise/Physical activities:	Plan for tomorrow:

Today's successes/Random thoughts:

Review of My Week

Things that really helped this week:

_____
_____
_____

Was/Were my goal(s) met?

_____
_____
_____

I'd like to work on this:

_____
_____
_____

Reminders of why I want to get to a healthier weight:

_____
_____
_____

Reminders of how my life is better already:

_____
_____
_____

MY WEIGHT:_____

MY SPACE

Don't deprive yourself.

"I realized that if I cut out things that I really enjoyed, I'd crave them. I love peanut butter, so when I was losing weight, I allowed myself to have a peanut butter sandwich 1 or 2 days a week. Finding that balance was important."

— David G.

About David: He started slimming down after reaching his highest weight of 260 when he was 16 and 5'9". David is now 20, weighs 195, and has grown to 5'11".

Habits before: "When I was at my worst, I would graze all day in the kitchen. Late at night and sometimes during the day, I would eat every snack I wanted until I was full. At meals, I would eat whatever I wanted, followed by dessert."

Turning point: What really did it was wanting to have a girlfriend. "I decided to do what-ever it took. I'd look at food and ask myself, 'What's more important — having this extra serving of something or getting in shape?'"

How he did it: "Overall healthy eating" and cutting back on unhealthy foods, along with exercise and avoiding eating at night. "Instead of going on diets and failing, I started making changes I could live with for the rest of my life." About once a week, he has a small dessert or special snack. He says, "It's better if you allow a small amount of treats fairly regularly. Then you don't binge and eat a bunch of them."

How he stays fit: David plays on his college racquetball team, does some toning exercises, and sometimes runs or goes for hikes.

How can you avoid depriving yourself without gaining?

Marie P.: "I allow myself one small treat per day, like a small piece of chocolate or a couple of cookies. That way, I get a little of what I'm craving without limiting myself too much."

Jayden L., who used to think there were "good foods and bad foods," now has "a higher-fat, more empty-calorie snack" about once a week.

Katie S.: "If I'm craving Doritos, I buy a single-serving bag to hit the spot."

Aaron T.'s strategy is to "think about what I eat before doing so. I can have chips with lunch if I have no cookie after dinner."

Jeana S. eats ice cream once a week or so, but only in a restaurant or store.

What's your plan for having occasional treats without going overboard?

_____

_____

_____

_____

try this:

AMBER M.'S EVERYDAY BANANA CREAM PIE

In a medium mixing bowl, prepare sugar-free instant vanilla pudding following the package directions (use fat-free or low-fat milk). Refrigerate for 10 to 15 minutes. Meanwhile, crush 4 graham crackers and divide the crumbs evenly among 4 single-serving bowls. Scoop $1/2$ c. pudding into each bowl and, just before eating, top each pudding with half a sliced banana.

my goal(s) for this week:

_____

_____

_____

Things that might trip me up:

_____

_____

_____

How I plan to deal with them:

_____

_____

_____

MY PLAN FOR EXERCISE/PHYSICAL ACTIVITY

Type of activity/length of time   **What I actually did**

Sunday:_____   _____

Monday:_____   _____

Tuesday:_____   _____

Wednesday:_____   _____

Thursday:_____   _____

Friday:_____   _____

Saturday:_____   _____

Daily Diary

Date: _____

Foods, beverages & snacks I had today:

	Food or beverage and amount	Hunger	Calories/Other	Feelings/Mood
MORNING				
AFTERNOON				
EVENING				
DAILY TOTAL				

Exercise/Physical activities:

Plan for tomorrow:

Today's successes/Random thoughts:

Daily Diary

Date: _____

Hunger: 1 = starving
2 = kind of hungry
3 = not hungry

Foods, beverages & snacks I had today:

	Food or beverage and amount	Hunger	Calories/Other	Feelings/Mood
MORNING				
AFTERNOON				
EVENING				
DAILY TOTAL				

Exercise/Physical activities:	Plan for tomorrow:

Today's successes/Random thoughts:

Daily Diary

Date:_____

Hunger: 1 = starving
2 = kind of hungry
3 = not hungry

Foods, beverages & snacks I had today:

	Food or beverage and amount	Hunger	Calories/Other	Feelings/Mood
MORNING				
AFTERNOON				
EVENING				
	DAILY TOTAL			

Exercise/Physical activities:	Plan for tomorrow:

Today's successes/Random thoughts:

Daily Diary

Date: _____

Foods, beverages & snacks I had today:

	Food or beverage and amount	Hunger	Calories/Other	Feelings/Mood
MORNING				
AFTERNOON				
EVENING				
DAILY TOTAL				

Exercise/Physical activities:

Plan for tomorrow:

Today's successes/Random thoughts:

Daily Diary

Date: _____

Hunger: 1 = starving
2 = kind of hungry
3 = not hungry

Foods, beverages & snacks I had today:

	Food or beverage and amount	Hunger	Calories/Other	Feelings/Mood
MORNING				
AFTERNOON				
EVENING				
DAILY TOTAL				

Exercise/Physical activities:

Plan for tomorrow:

Today's successes/Random thoughts:

Daily Diary

Date: _____

Hunger: 1 = starving
2 = kind of hungry
3 = not hungry

Foods, beverages & snacks I had today:

	Food or beverage and amount	Hunger	Calories/ Other	Feelings/Mood
MORNING				
AFTERNOON				
EVENING				
DAILY TOTAL				

Exercise/Physical activities:	Plan for tomorrow:

Today's successes/Random thoughts:

Daily Diary

Date:_____

Foods, beverages & snacks I had today:

	Food or beverage and amount	Hunger	Calories/Other	Feelings/Mood
MORNING				
AFTERNOON				
EVENING				
DAILY TOTAL				

Exercise/Physical activities:	Plan for tomorrow:

Today's successes/Random thoughts:

Review of My Week

◻ Things that really helped this week:

_____
_____
_____

◻ Was/Were my goal(s) met?

_____
_____
_____

◻ I'd like to work on this:

_____
_____
_____

◻ Reminders of why I want to get to a healthier weight:

_____
_____
_____

◻ Reminders of how my life is better already:

_____
_____
_____

MY WEIGHT:_____

MY SPACE

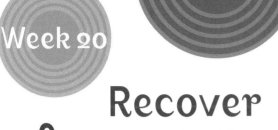

Recover from your slip-ups.

> "Once I slip, it's done. So instead of hounding myself, I try to find out why it happened. Then I try to figure out what I need to do to avoid it in the future."
>
> — Taylor S.

About Taylor: When Taylor hit his maximum weight of 250, he was 5'8". At 16, he started losing 100 pounds. He's now 19½, weighs 150, and is 5'9".

Habits before: "I was overweight from an unhealthy diet." His number one problem was snacking.

Turning point: "My uncle was in the hospital dying of cancer. That made me concerned about my own health. My main goal was to become healthy, rather than losing weight."

How he did it: It took Taylor more than 1½ years to lose 100 pounds. "Along with cutting out junk food and going on a low-sugar diet, I gave up meat, poultry, and snacks. Fish was my protein source." He also skateboarded, surfed, and played some basketball and football. He still avoids "junk food," but if he craves something, he has what he wants in moderation. He eats 5 or 6 times a day, has small portions, and has added meat back to his diet.

How he stays fit: "Right now, I'm trying to build my lean muscle through weight training, which I do 5 days a week, usually for 1 to 1½ hours. I take 2 days a week for rest."

How can YOU recover from your slips-ups?

Mike D.: "I let it go and just ease up at the next meal, because sometimes it's okay to give in."

Paula D.: "Sometimes I eat fattening foods like cookie batter and feel guilty. When that happens, I decide to look at the situation rationally. It's one slip-up, and it's not really *that* big a deal."

Katie S.: "If I gain a couple pounds, I tell myself, 'It's just a couple, and it's reversible.' Then I immediately get into action, assessing what made me gain."

What's your plan of action for slip-ups?

_____
_____
_____
_____
_____
_____

my goal(s) for this week:

_____
_____
_____

Things that might trip me up:

_____
_____
_____

How I plan to deal with them:

_____
_____
_____

MY PLAN FOR EXERCISE/PHYSICAL ACTIVITY

Type of activity/length of time

What I actually did

Sunday:_____   _____

Monday:_____   _____

Tuesday:_____   _____

Wednesday:_____   _____

Thursday:_____   _____

Friday:_____   _____

Saturday:_____   _____

Daily Diary

Date:_____

Hunger: 1 = starving
2 = kind of hungry
3 = not hungry

Foods, beverages & snacks I had today:

	Food or beverage and amount	Hunger	Calories/Other	Feelings/Mood
MORNING				
AFTERNOON				
EVENING				
	DAILY TOTAL			

Exercise/Physical activities:

Plan for tomorrow:

Today's successes/Random thoughts:

Daily Diary

Date: _____

Foods, beverages & snacks I had today:

	Food or beverage and amount	Hunger	Calories/Other	Feelings/Mood
MORNING				
AFTERNOON				
EVENING				
DAILY TOTAL				

Exercise/Physical activities:

Plan for tomorrow:

Today's successes/Random thoughts:

Daily Diary

Date:_____

Foods, beverages & snacks I had today:

	Food or beverage and amount	Hunger	Calories/Other	Feelings/Mood
MORNING				
AFTERNOON				
EVENING				
DAILY TOTAL				

Exercise/Physical activities:

Plan for tomorrow:

Today's successes/Random thoughts:

Daily Diary

Date: _____

Foods, beverages & snacks I had today:

Food or beverage and amount	Hunger	Calories/ Other	Feelings/Mood
DAILY TOTAL			

MORNING / AFTERNOON / EVENING

Exercise/Physical activities:	Plan for tomorrow:

Today's successes/Random thoughts:

Daily Diary

Date: _____

Foods, beverages & snacks I had today:

	Food or beverage and amount	Hunger	Calories/Other	Feelings/Mood
MORNING				
AFTERNOON				
EVENING				
DAILY TOTAL				

Exercise/Physical activities:

Plan for tomorrow:

Today's successes/Random thoughts:

Daily Diary

Date: _____

Hunger: 1 = starving
2 = kind of hungry
3 = not hungry

Foods, beverages & snacks I had today:

	Food or beverage and amount	Hunger	Calories/Other	Feelings/Mood
MORNING				
AFTERNOON				
EVENING				
DAILY TOTAL				

Exercise/Physical activities:	Plan for tomorrow:

Today's successes/Random thoughts:

Daily Diary

Date: _____

Hunger: 1 = starving
2 = kind of hungry
3 = not hungry

Foods, beverages & snacks I had today:

	Food or beverage and amount	Hunger	Calories/Other	Feelings/Mood
MORNING				
AFTERNOON				
EVENING				
DAILY TOTAL				

Exercise/Physical activities:

Plan for tomorrow:

Today's successes/Random thoughts:

Review of My Week

Things that really helped this week:

_____
_____
_____

Was/Were my goal(s) met?

_____
_____
_____

I'd like to work on this:

_____
_____
_____

Reminders of why I want to get to a healthier weight:

_____
_____
_____

Reminders of how my life is better already:

_____
_____
_____

MY WEIGHT:_____

MY SPACE

Make peace with your body.

> "I've realized that my imperfections are a part of me, and they always will be. What I can improve on, I work on to the best of my capabilities. What I can't improve, I have to accept."
>
> — Katie S.

About Katie: She started to become overweight when she was 12. By the time she was 18, Katie weighed 234 pounds. (She was 5'6½".) That's when she started slimming down to 140 pounds. She's 22 now and the same height.

Habits before: "Hamburgers were a staple of my diet," she says. "When my mom ridiculed me for being overweight, I ate more to upset her but hurt myself in the end."

Turning point: While on a trip, she met a woman who'd lost weight on a popular diet, which got Katie interested. When she saw how heavy she looked in the photos from the trip, she wanted to slim down even more so. "My parents had promised me a new wardrobe if I lost weight."

How she did it: "I lost the weight by exercising and by eating at Subway." (She chose subs made with lean meat, lots of veggies, and honey mustard.) She also cut back on fat and portions and counted calories. The only thing she gave up completely was doughnuts. Now, she says, "I rarely eat hamburgers. At restaurants, I take home half of my order and pick lighter items, like salads with the dressing on the side." And just about every day, she eats a few Hershey's Kisses.

How she stays fit: Every other day, she does cardio workouts involving a combination of walking and jogging for about 45 minutes. The other days, she does a shorter walk/run and uses weight machines for about half an hour.

try this:

ERIN C.'S PICKLE ROLL-UPS

Using a paper towel, pat dry the outside of a whole pickle, then spread some light cream cheese all over it. Wrap the pickle in a thin slice of ham and cut the whole thing into bite-sized circles.

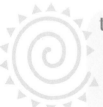

How can you make peace with your body?

Accept that there are some things you can't change. "Finally, after years of not being happy at my current weight, I realized that I wasn't meant to be a small person. As long as I'm toned up and I fit into my clothes, I need to be happy with myself." — Mary N.

Focus on your assets, not your flaws. Kristy C. says, "Maybe you have great hair or a fabulous smile or bright sparkly eyes or flawless skin."

Think about the things you really like about your appearance and about yourself in general.

_____

_____

_____

my goal(s) for this week:

_____

_____

_____

Things that might trip me up:	How I plan to deal with them:
_____	_____
_____	_____
_____	_____

MY PLAN FOR EXERCISE/PHYSICAL ACTIVITY

Type of activity/length of time	What I actually did
Sunday:_____	_____
Monday:_____	_____
Tuesday:_____	_____
Wednesday:_____	_____
Thursday:_____	_____
Friday:_____	_____
Saturday:_____	_____

Daily Diary

Date: _____

Foods, beverages & snacks I had today:

Food or beverage and amount	Hunger	Calories/ Other	Feelings/Mood

MORNING

AFTERNOON

EVENING

| DAILY TOTAL | | | |

Exercise/Physical activities:	Plan for tomorrow:

Today's successes/Random thoughts:

Daily Diary

Date:_____

Hunger: 1 = starving
2 = kind of hungry
3 = not hungry

Foods, beverages & snacks I had today:

	Food or beverage and amount	Hunger	Calories/Other	Feelings/Mood
MORNING				
AFTERNOON				
EVENING				
DAILY TOTAL				

Exercise/Physical activities:	Plan for tomorrow:

Today's successes/Random thoughts:

Daily Diary

Date: _____

Hunger: 1 = starving
2 = kind of hungry
3 = not hungry

Foods, beverages & snacks I had today:

	Food or beverage and amount	Hunger	Calories/Other	Feelings/Mood
MORNING				
AFTERNOON				
EVENING				
DAILY TOTAL				

Exercise/Physical activities:

Plan for tomorrow:

Today's successes/Random thoughts:

Daily Diary

Date: _____

Hunger: 1 = starving
2 = kind of hungry
3 = not hungry

Foods, beverages & snacks I had today:

	Food or beverage and amount	Hunger	Calories/ Other	Feelings/Mood
MORNING				
AFTERNOON				
EVENING				
DAILY TOTAL				

Exercise/Physical activities:	Plan for tomorrow:

Today's successes/Random thoughts:

Daily Diary

Date:_____

Foods, beverages & snacks I had today:

	Food or beverage and amount	Hunger	Calories/Other	Feelings/Mood
MORNING				
AFTERNOON				
EVENING				
DAILY TOTAL				

Exercise/Physical activities:	Plan for tomorrow:

Today's successes/Random thoughts:

Daily Diary

Date:_____

Hunger: 1 = starving
        2 = kind of hungry
        3 = not hungry

Foods, beverages & snacks I had today:

	Food or beverage and amount	Hunger	Calories/Other	Feelings/Mood
MORNING				
AFTERNOON				
EVENING				
DAILY TOTAL				

Exercise/Physical activities:	Plan for tomorrow:

Today's successes/Random thoughts:

Daily Diary

Date: _____

Hunger: 1 = starving
2 = kind of hungry
3 = not hungry

Foods, beverages & snacks I had today:

	Food or beverage and amount	Hunger	Calories/ Other	Feelings/Mood
MORNING				
AFTERNOON				
EVENING				
DAILY TOTAL				

Exercise/Physical activities:	Plan for tomorrow:

Today's successes/Random thoughts:

Review of My Week

Things that really helped this week:

_____
_____
_____

Was/Were my goal(s) met?

_____
_____
_____

I'd like to work on this:

_____
_____
_____

Reminders of why I want to get to a healthier weight:

_____
_____
_____

Reminders of how my life is better already:

_____
_____
_____

MY WEIGHT:_____

MY SPACE

If you start to gain, take action now, but don't panic.

> "One of the most important things I do to keep the weight off is that if I gain 5 pounds, I immediately lose it. I do something right away."
>
> — Zach G.

About Zach: The most Zach ever weighed was 283 pounds, when he was 5'9^1/$_2$" tall. He started losing more than 100 pounds when he was 14^1/$_2$. At 16^1/$_2$, he now weighs 178, and he's grown to 5'11^1/$_2$".

Habits before: "I used to eat like a machine. I could eat two bags of Twizzlers as a snack."

Turning point: Zach's mother had him watch some videos describing kids' summer weight camps, and he agreed to go to one of them.

How he did it: Zach lost about 40 pounds at Camp Pocono Trails, a summer weight camp, then lost the rest over the following school year. "The support of my friends and family was really important. I pretty much eat what I want, but portions are smaller. If I eat something fatty, I'll eat less later on." If Zach gains weight, he cuts back on the amount he eats.

How he stays fit: "Most days, I run 2 to 3 miles. I also play volleyball for 2 months out of the year."

How can you stop small weight gains?

Most of the teens weigh themselves regularly, but not fanatically, so they know whether their weight is beginning to creep up. They've learned that it's easier to deal with a small weight gain than to have to start all over again. If you lose weight but then start gaining some back, it can feel scary, and you might be tempted to take it off in an unhealthy way.

But it's normal for weight to creep up from time to time, and most of the teens have a healthy plan of action for when this happens. College student Tyler D., who keeps his weight within a 10-pound range, says, "If my weight's up, I cut back on snacking and drink more water." The teens' most common strategies for nipping small weight gains in the bud are exercising more, cutting back on snacks, going easy on sweets, and decreasing portions.

What's your plan of action if your weight creeps up?

_____
_____
_____
_____
_____

my goal(s) for this week:

_____
_____
_____

Things that might trip me up:

_____
_____
_____

How I plan to deal with them:

_____
_____
_____

MY PLAN FOR EXERCISE/PHYSICAL ACTIVITY

Type of activity/length of time

What I actually did

Sunday:_____   _____

Monday:_____   _____

Tuesday:_____   _____

Wednesday:_____   _____

Thursday:_____   _____

Friday:_____   _____

Saturday:_____   _____

Daily Diary

Date: _____

Hunger: 1 = starving
2 = kind of hungry
3 = not hungry

Foods, beverages & snacks I had today:

	Food or beverage and amount	Hunger	Calories/Other	Feelings/Mood
MORNING				
AFTERNOON				
EVENING				
DAILY TOTAL				

Exercise/Physical activities:

Plan for tomorrow:

Today's successes/Random thoughts:

Daily Diary

Date:_____

Hunger: 1 = starving
2 = kind of hungry
3 = not hungry

Foods, beverages & snacks I had today:

	Food or beverage and amount	Hunger	Calories/Other	Feelings/Mood
MORNING				
AFTERNOON				
EVENING				
	DAILY TOTAL			

Exercise/Physical activities:	Plan for tomorrow:

Today's successes/Random thoughts:

Daily Diary

Date: _____

Hunger: 1 = starving
2 = kind of hungry
3 = not hungry

Foods, beverages & snacks I had today:

	Food or beverage and amount	Hunger	Calories/Other	Feelings/Mood
MORNING				
AFTERNOON				
EVENING				
DAILY TOTAL				

Exercise/Physical activities:	Plan for tomorrow:

Today's successes/Random thoughts:

Daily Diary

Date: _____

Hunger: 1 = starving
2 = kind of hungry
3 = not hungry

Foods, beverages & snacks I had today:

	Food or beverage and amount	Hunger	Calories/Other	Feelings/Mood
MORNING				
AFTERNOON				
EVENING				
	DAILY TOTAL			

Exercise/Physical activities:	Plan for tomorrow:

Today's successes/Random thoughts:

Daily Diary

Date:_____

Foods, beverages & snacks I had today:

	Food or beverage and amount	Hunger	Calories/ Other	Feelings/Mood
MORNING				
AFTERNOON				
EVENING				
DAILY TOTAL				

Exercise/Physical activities:	Plan for tomorrow:

Today's successes/Random thoughts:

Daily Diary

Date: _____

Hunger: 1 = starving
2 = kind of hungry
3 = not hungry

Foods, beverages & snacks I had today:

	Food or beverage and amount	Hunger	Calories/Other	Feelings/Mood
MORNING				
AFTERNOON				
EVENING				
DAILY TOTAL				

Exercise/Physical activities:	Plan for tomorrow:

Today's successes/Random thoughts:

Daily Diary

Date: _____

Foods, beverages & snacks I had today:

	Food or beverage and amount	Hunger	Calories/Other	Feelings/Mood
MORNING				
AFTERNOON				
EVENING				
DAILY TOTAL				

Exercise/Physical activities:

Plan for tomorrow:

Today's successes/Random thoughts:

Review of My Week

Things that really helped this week:

_____

_____

_____

Was/Were my goal(s) met?

_____

_____

_____

I'd like to work on this:

_____

_____

_____

Reminders of why I want to get to a healthier weight:

_____

_____

_____

Reminders of how my life is better already:

_____

_____

_____

MY WEIGHT:_____

MY SPACE

Week 23

Get rid of "diet thinking."

"I don't think of what I do as a diet — it's a change in lifestyle. It is not temporary. I'm happy with who I am now, and I don't want to go back."

— Joyelle T.

About Joyelle: "I was overweight my whole life. At 14, I weighed 215 and felt like an outcast." At 14½, she began a gradual process of losing 55 pounds. She's now 17, weighs 160, and is 5'3".

Habits before: Joyelle thinks the number one reason she became overweight is because of a family tendency — her parents and her brother are overweight. Also, her portions were too big, she snacked too often, and she didn't get enough exercise.

Turning point: "I was embarrassed by my size and wanted to be healthy." She'd lost some weight on her own but got stuck at 185. One day, she saw herself in a mirror and said, "I can't do this anymore."

How she did it: Joyelle lost her first 30 pounds on a low-fat diet that she and her parents came up with. Then she joined Jenny Craig, which helped her lose another 25 pounds. She adds, "I stopped eating fast food and began walking and running." Joyelle's success motivated her father to lose more than 100 pounds. She still avoids high-fat, high-sugar, and fast foods. And about once a month, she treats herself to Chinese food or "grandma's lasagna."

How she stays fit: "I do Tae Bo for 30 minutes every day. I also have volleyball practice 5 days a week for 2 hours."

How can YOU get rid of "diet thinking"?

Like Joyelle, other teens say they've shifted away from "dieting" to making changes they can live with for a lifetime.

Rebecca M.: "People who are on diets see it as only a temporary thing and then go back to the way they used to eat. But a lifestyle is permanent. I choose to eat the way I do and exercise because I never want to look the way I used to. I've found foods that are healthy *and* good to eat, so I don't feel like I'm just eating this way temporarily."

Make a list of changes you've made or would like to make in your eating and exercise habits that you feel you can keep doing — for instance, eating breakfast, having at least five fruits and vegetables each day, or walking for half an hour 5 days a week.

_____
_____
_____
_____

my goal(s) for this week:

_____
_____
_____

Things that might trip me up:

_____
_____
_____

How I plan to deal with them:

_____
_____
_____

MY PLAN FOR EXERCISE/PHYSICAL ACTIVITY

Type of activity/length of time   What I actually did

Sunday:_____   _____

Monday:_____   _____

Tuesday:_____   _____

Wednesday:_____   _____

Thursday:_____   _____

Friday:_____   _____

Saturday:_____   _____

Daily Diary

Date: _____

Foods, beverages & snacks I had today:

	Food or beverage and amount	Hunger	Calories/Other	Feelings/Mood
MORNING				
AFTERNOON				
EVENING				
	DAILY TOTAL			

Exercise/Physical activities:

Plan for tomorrow:

Today's successes/Random thoughts:

Daily Diary

Date: _____

Foods, beverages & snacks I had today:

	Food or beverage and amount	Hunger	Calories/Other	Feelings/Mood
MORNING				
AFTERNOON				
EVENING				
	DAILY TOTAL			

Exercise/Physical activities:	Plan for tomorrow:

Today's successes/Random thoughts:

Daily Diary

Date: _____

Hunger: 1 = starving
2 = kind of hungry
3 = not hungry

Foods, beverages & snacks I had today:

	Food or beverage and amount	Hunger	Calories/Other	Feelings/Mood
MORNING				
AFTERNOON				
EVENING				
DAILY TOTAL				

Exercise/Physical activities:

Plan for tomorrow:

Today's successes/Random thoughts:

Daily Diary

Date:_____

Foods, beverages & snacks I had today:

	Food or beverage and amount	Hunger	Calories/Other	Feelings/Mood
MORNING				
AFTERNOON				
EVENING				
	DAILY TOTAL			

Exercise/Physical activities:	Plan for tomorrow:
Today's successes/Random thoughts:	

Daily Diary

Date: _____

Hunger: 1 = starving
2 = kind of hungry
3 = not hungry

Foods, beverages & snacks I had today:

	Food or beverage and amount	Hunger	Calories/Other	Feelings/Mood
MORNING				
AFTERNOON				
EVENING				
DAILY TOTAL				

Exercise/Physical activities:	Plan for tomorrow:

Today's successes/Random thoughts:

Daily Diary

Date: _____

Hunger: 1 = starving
2 = kind of hungry
3 = not hungry

Foods, beverages & snacks I had today:

	Food or beverage and amount	Hunger	Calories/ Other	Feelings/Mood
MORNING				
AFTERNOON				
EVENING				
	DAILY TOTAL			

Exercise/Physical activities:	Plan for tomorrow:

Today's successes/Random thoughts:

Daily Diary

Date: _____

Hunger: 1 = starving
2 = kind of hungry
3 = not hungry

Foods, beverages & snacks I had today:

	Food or beverage and amount	Hunger	Calories/Other	Feelings/Mood
MORNING				
AFTERNOON				
EVENING				
DAILY TOTAL				

Exercise/Physical activities:	Plan for tomorrow:

Today's successes/Random thoughts:

Review of My Week

Things that really helped this week:

_____
_____
_____

Was/Were my goal(s) met?

_____
_____
_____

I'd like to work on this:

_____
_____
_____

Reminders of why I want to get to a healthier weight:

_____
_____
_____

Reminders of how my life is better already:

_____
_____
_____

MY WEIGHT:_____

MY SPACE

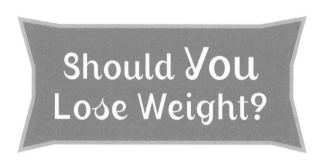

Should You Lose Weight?

To determine whether you're overweight, health professionals use a special math formula to come up with what's called your body mass index, or BMI. You can find out if your BMI puts you in the overweight category by checking with your doctor or visiting this Web site: http://apps.nccd.cdc.gov/dnpabmi/Calculator.aspx. Being overweight means that you have an excessively high amount of body fat for your height, age, and sex.

If you're still growing and you're not very overweight, you may not acually need to lose pounds because you can "grow into your weight" through physical activity and healthy eating. However, if you've finished growing and/or you're very overweight, gradual weight loss is probably appropriate. The best way to find out whether you should be losing weight or waiting until you grow into your weight is to check with a physician.

If weight loss is recommended, a safe rate of slimming down is 1 to 2 pounds per week. If you lose more than that, your body may start losing too much muscle tissue along with the fat, and that's not healthy. If you're hungry all the time, that's a sign that your diet is too strict and you're losing weight too fast.

Doing the Math

To go from being overweight to a healthy weight, you need to eat fewer calories than your body uses each day or increase your physical activity so that you burn more calories than you eat. The vast majority of the teens I interviewed said they did both.

Calories measure the energy we get from eating three different nu-

trients in foods: carbohydrates, protein, and fat. (The other nutrients —
vitamins, minerals, and water — provide no calories.) Carbohydrates
and protein provide about 4 calories per gram, while fat supplies 9 calories per gram. Alcohol, which is not a nutrient, provides approximately
7 calories per gram. (A gram is about one thirtieth of an ounce.) Since
fat has more than double the calories of the other nutrients, fatty foods
are more likely to cause a weight gain than are lower-fat foods.

It's hard to say how many total calories per day you'll need to maintain your weight because it depends on so many different things. Physical activity is a big part of the picture — the part over which you have
the most control. The more physically active you are, the more calories
you need. Taller and heavier teens generally need more calories than
shorter and lighter teens of the same age and activity level. Muscle tissue
burns more calories than fat tissue, so if you're muscular, you'll probably
burn more calories than out-of-shape teens of the same age and size.
When you're going through a growth spurt, your calorie needs increase.
Guys generally need more calories than girls of the same age.

If you're a girl trying to lose weight on your own, you shouldn't eat
fewer than 1,600 calories per day, because you'll have a hard time getting
the nutrients you need to be healthy. A number of experts feel the minimum for guys is about 1,800 calories per day. Even at these acceptable
calorie levels, it might be wise to take a multivitamin/mineral supple-
ment. Again, check with your doctor.

How long will it take to get to your desired weight? Let's say you're a
16-year-old girl who's 5'5" and weighs 175 pounds, and you want to get
down to 140. We'll assume that you're not very active and that you're
staying at your current weight while eating 2,600 calories a day. If you
cut your daily calorie level to 2,100 calories, you'll be eating 500 calories
less each day than you're burning. Multiply that 500 calories by 7 days in
a week, and you get 3,500 calories. Since 3,500 is the approximate number of calories in a pound of body weight, you should lose about 1
pound per week on a 2,100-calorie plan. On a 1,600-calorie plan, you'll
lose around 2 pounds per week.

As your body becomes smaller, weight loss tends to become a bit
slower, because your smaller body just doesn't need as many calories as

your bigger body did. If things seem too slow, you may choose to step up your physical activity, but don't overdo it.

How Many Calories for How Much Exercise?

The following chart shows how many calories a 154-pound adult burns by doing different types of physical activity. If you're lighter, you'll burn fewer calories; if you're heavier, you'll burn more. Teens who are 15 to 16 or older probably burn about the same number of calories as adults of the same weight for any particular activity done for the same length of time. Younger teens probably burn more calories than adults of the same weight.

APPROXIMATE CALORIES BURNED PER HOUR	
MODERATE PHYSICAL ACTIVITIES	
Hiking	370
Light gardening/yard work	330
Dancing	330
Golf (walking and carrying clubs)	330
Bicycling (<10 mph)	290
Walking (3.5 mph)	280
Weightlifting (general light workout)	220
Stretching	180
VIGOROUS PHYSICAL ACTIVITIES	
Running/jogging (5 mph)	590
Bicycling (>10 mph)	590
Swimming (slow freestyle laps)	510
Aerobics	480
Walking, brisk (4.5 mph)	460
Heavy yard work (like chopping wood)	440
Weightlifting (vigorous effort)	440
Basketball (vigorous)	440

Source: U.S. Department of Health and Human Services and U.S. Department of Agriculture, Dietary Guidelines for Americans, 2005.
Note: The calorie values listed above include calories used by the activity as well as calories used for normal body functions. For more on calorie expenditure for various activities, go to www.mypyramidtracker.gov or www.caloriesperhour.com.

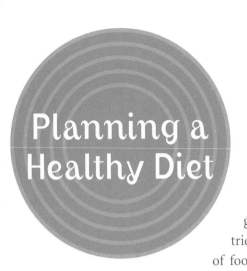

Planning a Healthy Diet

Some of the teens used a "food pyramid" to guide their everyday eating choices. In school, you've probably learned about this concept, now called MyPyramid — a government-sponsored guide that groups foods according to their nutrient content and indicates the amount of food from each group you should eat each day to be healthy. After trying several fad diets that didn't work, Jeana S. began her 22-pound weight loss journey by becoming more active, eating six mini-meals a day, packing her own lunch, and following the food pyramid. Angel W. says that following the food pyramid helps her keep off 65 pounds.

To show you an example of what a healthy weight loss plan might include, I've provided the chart below, based on recommendations from MyPyramid, with guidelines for a 1,600-, 1,800-, and 2,000-calorie food plan. (For more detailed information about the food groups and to determine how other foods "count," go to www.mypyramid.gov. Watch for MyPyramid's new online menu planner to help you create meals to meet your personal MyPyramid food-group recommendations.)

Daily Eating Plan

The 1,600-calorie plan is for girls only. The 1,800- and 2,000-calorie plans are for girls or boys. (If you're very active or "growing into your weight," you may need more calories than this.) The plans are designed with overweight 12- to 18-year-olds in mind, who have been given their physician's okay to follow such plans. (If you're a vegetarian or have any medical conditions, such as diabetes, you should seek the help of a registered dietitian to make your meal plans to ensure they meet your nutrient needs.) Be aware that the foods within any one group do not necessarily have the same number of calories. For instance, 1/2 cup of raisins has about 250 calories, while 1 cup of grapes has roughly 110 calories. It's important to eat a variety of foods within all the food groups.

FOOD GROUP	FOOD CHOICES	1,600-calorie	1,800-calorie	2,000-calorie
GRAINS[1] (see page 248)		5 oz.	6 oz.	6 oz.
	AMOUNT THAT COUNTS AS 1 oz.			
	1 slice bread			
	1/2 c. cooked pasta or rice or cooked cereal			
	1 packet instant oatmeal			
	1 oz. dried pasta or rice			
	1 small muffin (2 1/2" diameter)			
	1 small biscuit (2" diameter)			
	1/2 English muffin			
	1 small pita bread (4" diameter)			
	1 c. ready-to-eat flake cereal			
	1 mini-bagel or 1/4 of a 4-oz. bagel			
	5 whole-wheat crackers			
	4 graham cracker squares (2 rectangles)			
	7 square or round crackers			
	1 pancake (4 1/2")			
	3 c. popped popcorn (without butter)			
	6" flour or corn tortilla			
	1 toaster waffle			
VEGETABLES[2] (see page 249)		2 c.	2 1/2 c.	2 1/2 c.
	AMOUNT THAT COUNTS AS 1 CUP			
	1 c. raw or cooked vegetables, such as chopped broccoli, green peas, cauliflower, shredded cabbage, squash, green beans, onions, cucumbers, mushrooms			
	2 c. raw leafy greens, such as lettuce or spinach			
	1 c. vegetable juice, such as V 8			
	3 broccoli spears			
	2 medium carrots or 12 baby carrots			
	1 c. cooked dried beans or peas, such as black beans, chickpeas, kidney beans, or soybeans			
	1 c. or 1 large ear corn			
	1 medium white potato (2 1/2–3" diameter)			
	1 large sweet potato (2 1/4" diameter)			
	1 large tomato			
	2 large celery stalks			

FOOD GROUP	FOOD CHOICES	1,600-calorie	1,800-calorie	2,000-calorie
	1 large green or red bell pepper			
	1 c. salsa			
	½ c. spaghetti sauce			
FRUITS[3] (see page 249)		1½ c.	1½ c.	2 c.
	AMOUNT THAT COUNTS AS 1 CUP			
	½ large or 1 small apple			
	1 c. applesauce (no sugar added)			
	1 c. sliced or 1 large banana			
	1 c. diced cantaloupe or melon balls			
	1 c. grapes			
	1 medium grapefruit			
	1 large orange			
	1 c. mandarin oranges, drained			
	1 c. sliced/diced or 1 large peach			
	1 c. sliced/diced or 1 medium pear			
	1 c. pineapple chunks			
	3 medium or 2 large plums			
	1 c. sliced or 8 large strawberries			
	1"-thick wedge watermelon			
	½ c. dried fruit, such as raisins, apricots, or plums			
	1 c. unsweetened fruit juice			
MILK[4] (see page 249)		3 c.	3 c.	3 c.
	AMOUNT THAT COUNTS AS 1 C., PREFERABLY FAT-FREE OR LOW-FAT			
	1 c. or 1 half-pt. carton milk			
	½ c. evaporated milk			
	1 c. yogurt			
	1½ oz. cheddar, Swiss, or mozzarella cheese			
	⅓ c. shredded cheese			
	2 oz. processed cheese, such as American			
	½ c. ricotta cheese			
	AMOUNT THAT COUNTS AS ½ OF A MILK SERVING			
	1 c. cottage cheese			
	½ c. pudding, made with milk			
	½ c. frozen yogurt			
	¾ c. ice cream			

FOOD GROUP	FOOD CHOICES	1,600-calorie	1,800-calorie	2,000-calorie
MEAT & BEANS[5] [see page 249] (*Dried beans can be counted either as vegetables or in the meat and beans group, but you can't count a single portion as both.)		5 oz.	5 oz.	6 oz.

AMOUNT THAT COUNTS AS 1 oz.

1 oz. cooked lean beef, pork, or ham

1 oz. cooked chicken or turkey, without skin

1 sandwich slice of turkey or lean ham

1 oz. cooked fish or shellfish

1 egg

1/2 oz. nuts, such as 12 almonds, 24 pistachios, or 7 walnut halves

1/2 oz. seeds, hulled and roasted, such as sunflower or pumpkin

1 Tbsp. peanut butter or almond butter

1/4 c. cooked dried peas or beans, such as baked beans; refried beans; lentils; black, kidney, pinto, or white beans; chickpeas; or split peas*

1/4 c. tofu (about 2 ounces)

1/2 soyburger patty

1/4 c. roasted soybeans

2 Tbsp. hummus

1/2 fat-free or low-fat hot dog

OILS[6] [see page 249]		5 tsp.	5 tsp.	5 tsp.

AMOUNT THAT COUNTS AS 1 tsp.

1 tsp. vegetable oil (corn, canola, safflower, soybean, olive, sunflower)

1 tsp. soft margarine (with no trans fat)

1 Tbsp. low-fat mayonnaise

2 Tbsp. light salad dressing

1 Tbsp. Italian salad dressing

8 large, ripe olives

CALORIES LEFT FOR "EXTRAS"[7] [see page 249]	130	195	265

1. At least half your choices should come from whole-grain cereals, breads, crackers, rice, or pasta. When possible, make choices from low-fat items and those that don't have added sugar.

2. Vary your veggies so that you have several subgroups each day, such as dark green, orange, leafy green, starchy (corn, potatoes, green peas), and dried beans.

3. In general, 1 c. fruit or 100% fruit juice can be considered as 1 c. from the fruit group. Make most choices fruits, not juices. Fruits may be fresh, frozen, or canned (drained), but avoid those packed in heavy syrup. Try to eat a variety of fruits.

4. The list has foods that count as a 1-c. (or ½-c.) milk serving in terms of calcium but not necessarily in terms of calories, so check labels for calorie content. When using sweetened products, select those with no-calorie sweeteners like sucralose and aspartame, rather than products with added sugar, dextrose, or corn syrup.

5. Avoid fatty meats and high-fat lunch meats. Choose fish and dried beans frequently.

6. Oils are not really considered a food group, but you need some for good health. Be sure to count oils used in food preparation.

7. If you choose the lowest-fat and no-sugar-added items in each food group, you may have some calories left to "spend" on extras such as solid fats (like butter), sauces, syrup, jelly, candy, sugar, regular salad dressing, or a dessert. You can also spend the extra calories on additional portions from any of the other food groups or on a higher-calorie version of a food than appears in the group — a higher-fat meat such as a hamburger patty, for example. Or you can "save up" your extra calories from one day to the next. For instance, you might save your extra calories for 2 days to spend on a piece of pie.

Source: Adapted from www.mypyramid.gov, U.S. Department of Agriculture, Center for Nutrition Policy and Promotion.

Foods You Don't Have to "Count"

Reasonable amounts of the following foods can be used without "counting" them (check labels to make sure specific items have few or no calories):

Beverages
water
sugar-free soft drinks
carbonated or sparkling water
black coffee or tea (go easy on caffeine, especially later in the day)
sugar-free drink mixes
fat-free bouillon or broth (preferably reduced sodium)

Flavoring agents
sugar substitutes, such as sucralose (Splenda), aspartame (Equal), and saccharin (Sweet'N Low)
low-calorie butter-flavoring products, such as Butter Buds

lemon or lime juice

flavoring extracts, such as vanilla and almond

herbs and spices

horseradish

soy or Worcestershire sauce

mustard

vinegar

garlic

Miscellaneous

nonstick cooking spray

sugar-free, low-calorie gelatin dessert (no more than 1 envelope
per day)

sugar-free gum

unsweetened pickles

Saving Calories by Shaving Fat

Take a look at all the calories you can save by simply substituting lower-fat foods for similar items that are higher in fat. Any one of these might not look like a big calorie saving, but when you add them up, the net saving in one day is about 550 calories — without ever "dieting." If you save that many calories every day, you'll lose about 1 pound a week, quite painlessly.

SUBSTITUTE THIS	FOR THIS	CALORIES YOU'LL SAVE
English muffin with 1 Tbsp. jam	1 large blueberry muffin	197
1 oz. low-fat cheddar cheese	1 oz. regular cheddar cheese	65
3 oz. cooked extra-lean hamburger (5% fat)	3 oz. cooked regular hamburger (25% fat)	88
1 c. fat-free milk	1 c. whole milk	56
1 c. low-fat frozen yogurt	1 c. regular ice cream	70
3 oz. roasted chicken, skinless	3 oz. fried chicken (leg meat, with skin)	72

Note: You can easily do your own searches and comparisons by going to the USDA National Nutrient Database at www.nal.usda.gov/fnic/foodcomp/search/index.html.

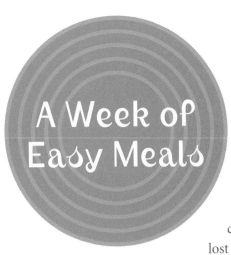

A Week of Easy Meals

To show you examples of actual meals and snacks for a healthy 1,800-calorie plan, I've provided the following menus for a week of easy breakfasts, lunches, dinners, and snacks. They're loosely based on the MyPyramid guidelines and include some ideas from the teens who lost weight and kept it off.

Day 1

Breakfast

2 high-fiber frozen waffles, such as the Kashi GoLean brand

$^1/_2$ c. fresh blueberries to top the waffles

2 Tbsp. reduced-calorie syrup drizzled over the blueberries

1 c. fat-free milk

Lunch

AARON T.'S QUICK-MEAL SALAD Place the following in a big plastic zipper-lock bag and shake gently.

2 c. ready-made salad greens

$^1/_4$ c. cherry tomatoes

2 oz. cooked turkey breast, cubed

$^1/_4$ c. chickpeas

2 Tbsp. balsamic vinegar

1 tsp. salad oil, such as olive or corn oil

1 tsp. Dijon mustard

1 tsp. honey

Salt-free Italian seasoning blend, to taste

1 oz. fat-free croutons

$^1/_2$ c. grapes

1 c. fat-free milk

Dinner

SANDRA D.'S SALMON STIR-FRY Place the following in a large frying pan coated with nonstick spray, then cover and cook over medium-high heat, stirring occasionally, until vegetables are cooked.

1 c. bite-sized pieces of broccoli

$^1/_2$ c. pea pods

$^1/_2$ c. sliced onions

2 tsp. sesame oil

1 Tbsp. store-bought stir-fry sauce

2 oz. cooked salmon, broken into chunks

Lemon or lime juice, to taste

1 c. cooked brown rice

1 c. fat-free milk

1 c. diced watermelon

Snacks

1 large orange

3 c. popped popcorn

2 tsp. soft margarine, melted (drizzle over popcorn)

Day 2

Breakfast

WES G.'S PEANUT BUTTER–BANANA ROLL-UP (see page 32 for directions)

1 whole-wheat tortilla (6" diameter)

2 Tbsp. reduced-fat peanut butter

$^1/_2$ large banana, sliced thin

1 light yogurt smoothie, such as Dannon Light & Fit (7 oz.)

Lunch

1 slice restaurant cheese pizza (from a 12" pizza)

1–2 c. mixed salad greens

2 Tbsp. light Italian dressing

1 medium pear

1 c. fat-free milk

Dinner

3 oz. roasted chicken breast, without skin

1 large sweet potato, baked

1 c. steamed broccoli

Whole-wheat dinner roll

2 tsp. soft margarine

1 c. fat-free milk

Snacks

1 baked soft pretzel (2 oz.)

1 snack cup (4 oz.) fruit-flavored applesauce (sweetened with no-calorie sweetener)

$^1/_2$ c. soft serve ice cream

Day 3

Breakfast

ETHAN Q.'S YOGURT PARFAIT (see page 73 for directions)

1 c. light nonfat berry or vanilla yogurt

$^1/_4$ c. Grape-Nuts cereal

$^1/_2$ c. fresh raspberries

1 slice whole-wheat toast

1 tsp. soft margarine

Lunch

OPEN-FACED SANDWICH

$^1/_2$ whole-wheat bagel

2 oz. deli turkey breast

1 slice provolone cheese

Lettuce leaves

2 slices tomato

1 Tbsp. low-fat mayonnaise

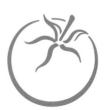

1 oz. baked potato chips

12 raw baby carrots

Water or diet soda

Dinner

SPAGHETTI WITH MEATBALLS

1 c. cooked whole-wheat spaghetti

$^1/_2$ c. spaghetti sauce

4 small meatballs (2 oz. total)

1 Tbsp. grated Parmesan cheese

SPINACH SALAD

2 c. spinach

Red onion slices

2 Tbsp. light salad dressing

1 c. fat-free milk

Snacks

ORANGE FROSTY SHAKE

Combine in a blender:

$^1/_4$ c. orange juice concentrate

$^3/_4$ c. fat-free milk

$^1/_2$ tsp. vanilla extract

3–4 ice cubes

Sugar substitute, to taste

24 pistachio nuts, preferably unsalted

1 fruit snack cup (4 oz.)

Day 4

Breakfast

2 mini or $^1/_2$ of a 4-oz. cinnamon raisin bagel

$^1/_2$ c. light ricotta cheese, topped with 2 Tbsp. apple butter (Try some
on the bagels, and eat the rest with a spoon)

1 c. diced cantaloupe

Lunch

TUNA SALAD SANDWICH
- 1 foil-pack tuna (3 oz.)
- 2 Tbsp. low-fat mayonnaise
- 2 slices whole-wheat bread
- 1 large tomato, cut into slices

1 c. fat-free milk

Dinner

WES G.'S RICE, BEANS, AND SALSA Layer rice, beans, and salsa in a microwavable bowl, then top with cheese, and microwave until hot.
- 1 c. cooked brown rice
- $1/2$ c. fat-free refried beans
- $1/4$ c. salsa
- $1/3$ c. grated reduced-fat Mexican-blend cheese

Raw Veggies
$1/2$ large green or red bell pepper, cut into strips
1 celery stalk
Water or diet soda

Snacks

TRAIL MIX
- $1/4$ c. dried fruit
- $1/2$ c. roasted soybeans
- 2 Tbsp. chocolate chips

ZACH G.'S MOCK ICE CREAM SANDWICH
(see page 233 for directions)
- 1 graham cracker
- 2 Tbsp. fat-free whipped topping

8 large strawberries

Day 5

Breakfast

1 low-fat peanut butter granola bar

BANANA SHAKE

Combine in a blender:

1 c. fat-free milk

1 large frozen banana, broken into chunks

1 tsp. vanilla extract

No-calorie sweetener, to taste (optional)

Lunch

10 reduced-fat Triscuit crackers

$^1/_4$ c. hummus (spread on the Triscuits)

1 c. bite-sized pieces of raw vegetables, such as broccoli or cauliflower

2 Tbsp. light Ranch dressing for the veggies

1 pudding cup (4 oz.)

1 c. fat-free milk

Dinner

ONION AND SWISS BURGER

1 whole-wheat hamburger bun

3-oz. broiled lean-beef patty

1 slice reduced-fat Swiss cheese

$^1/_4$ c. sliced onions, sautéed in nonstick pan

1 large corn on the cob

2 tsp. soft margarine for corn

COLESLAW

1 c. shredded cabbage

2 Tbsp. store-bought reduced-fat coleslaw dressing

Water or diet soda

Snacks

1 c. Cheerios with $^1/_2$ c. fat-free milk

$^1/_2$ c. grapes

Day 6

Breakfast

BREAKFAST BURRITO
  1 whole-wheat tortilla (6" diameter)
  1 egg, scrambled
  ^{1}/4 c. canned black beans, preferably salt-free
  2 Tbsp. salsa
  ^{1}/4 c. grated reduced-fat cheddar cheese

^{1}/2 c. calcium-fortified orange juice

Lunch

PEANUT BUTTER AND JELLY SANDWICH
  2 slices whole-wheat bread
  2 Tbsp. peanut butter
  1 Tbsp. jelly

1 large banana
1 c. fat-free milk

Dinner

ZACH G.'S PITA PIZZA (see page 23 for directions)
  1 whole-wheat pita (6" diameter), split in half
  ^{1}/4 c. spaghetti sauce
  ^{1}/3 c. grated part-skim mozzarella cheese

1 c. grape tomatoes and cucumber slices
1 c. fat-free milk
2 Tbsp. chocolate syrup (mix into milk)

Snacks

1 small muffin
^{1}/2 oz. sunflower seeds, preferably unsalted
^{1}/2 c. fresh pineapple chunks
JORGEY W.'S LOW-FAT FRIES (see page 113 for directions)
  1 medium white potato

Day 7

Breakfast

1 packet instant oatmeal, prepared with 1 c. fat-free milk

$1/4$ c. raisins (sprinkle on top of or mix into oatmeal)

$1/2$ oz. (about $2^1/2$ Tbsp.) sliced almonds (sprinkle on top of oatmeal)

Lunch

2 fast-food soft-shell tacos

Fast-food side salad

2 Tbsp. light salad dressing

1 small apple

Water or diet soda

Dinner

1 package single-serving macaroni and cheese, such as Kraft Easy Mac

1 c. cooked green peas

$1/2$ c. mandarin orange slices

1 c. fat-free milk

Snacks

$1/2$ c. frozen yogurt

2 Tbsp. caramel topping (drizzle over yogurt)

1 hard-cooked egg

5 whole-wheat crackers

$3/4$ oz. reduced-fat cheese

1 celery stalk

Acknowledgments

My deep appreciation goes to the teens, their parents, and the many experts who provided information for *Weight Loss Confidential* and the *Weight Loss Confidential Journal.* Thanks, too, to the countless friends, teachers, counselors, weight programs, educators, colleagues, Web sites, and other organizations that helped me recruit young people for these books. For reviewing material in the journal, my special thanks goes to teen-weight expert Kerri Boutelle, Ph.D., associate professor of pediatrics and psychiatry at the University of California, San Diego; Jamie Stang, Ph.D., an adolescent nutrition expert at the University of Minnesota; and my daughter, Julia, for her creative, teen-friendly editing help.

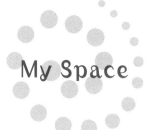

My Space

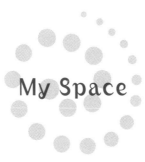

My Space

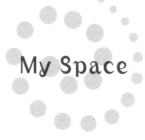

My Space